$7.50

MANUAL OF
PEDIATRIC PHYSICAL DIAGNOSIS

Manual of PEDIATRIC Physical Diagnosis

by

LEWIS A. BARNESS, M.D.

Professor of Pediatrics
University of South Florida College of Medicine
Tampa, Florida

Fourth Edition

YEAR BOOK MEDICAL PUBLISHERS • INC.

35 EAST WACKER DRIVE • CHICAGO 60601

Library of Congress Catalog Card Number: 79-150740

International Standard Book Number: 0-8151-0492-8

Reprinted, September 1960

Second edition, 1961

Third edition, 1966

Reprinted, April 1968

Reprinted, January 1971

Fourth edition, November 1972

Reprinted, April 1973

Reprinted, May 1974

To my first pediatricians,
my mother and father

Preface to the Fourth Edition

A new edition of this manual was felt to be necessary to add several diagnostic findings and to include some of the newer useful developmental information.

Many readers have written to help correct and revise the manuscript. As always, the students have been constructively critical.

Dr. Edward Shaw of San Francisco, in particular, has written many worthwhile aids in physical diagnosis. Most of these are included, with sincere appreciation.

Some diagnosticians in the past several years have written suggesting that the physical examination should be downgraded in pediatrics, because most of the pediatric diagnoses can be made from histories or laboratory examination. I believe this attitude is deplorable and only partly true. The physical examination is responsible not only for making diagnoses but also for confirming suspected diagnoses. The laboratory remains a tool which needs to be corrected by history, physical examination, and common sense.

When the third edition of this book appeared, the threat of the computer to the physician was mentioned. Since that time a computer-assisted diagnosis system in pediatrics has been developed. Experience with computers in medicine thus far seems to indicate that computers cannot replace the physician. Indeed, the opposite seems true. The computer requires accurate input. This must be derived from the physician, who can take an accurate history and perform and interpret correctly a complete physical examination.

The advent of computer-assisted diagnosis, however, has caused the elimination of the appendix relating to particular physical characteristics of rare syndromes, which appeared in the first three editions. The number of such

syndromes, also, would make such a section too long for
this book.

One persistent criticism which still goes uncorrected
is the large amount of information included. Attempts at
simplification have been made. For the novice I apologize
that the book is not simpler, but I hope the complexities
included will help develop a vocabulary more quickly.
For those who see mainly normal children, fundamental
grounding still is most easily accomplished by the study
of the abnormal.

My sincere thanks to all those mentioned in previous
editions, especially Drs. Mellman, Oski, Morrow and
Schmidt, to Dr. Thomas Tedesco for the diagrams, to
those who have allowed me to use material from their
published works, and, as always, to my severest critics,
Elaine, Carol, Laura, and Joe. Again, my secretary,
Mrs. Verdie Thomas, has put up with multiple chores,
for which I am grateful.

L. A. B.

Preface to the First Edition

This manual originated several years ago as a series of mimeographed notes to second-year medical students at the University of Pennsylvania Medical School.
Each year, the notes on pediatric physical examination
expanded as no suitable text for the course was found.

Three years ago Dean John McK. Mitchell and Dr.
Paul György suggested that this material be gathered together in book form. The material has been further expanded for this purpose.

Physical examination is a discipline learned by observing and practicing; my teachers have supplied the op-
portunity for these observations. Especially among these
are included Dr. Paul György who taught me many tricks
and fine points of examination of children; Drs. Charles
Janeway and Sydney Gellis who taught me the approach to

the pediatric patient; Dr. Bronson Crothers who taught an inimitable approach to the pediatric patient with neurological disorders; seven classes of medical students who gave free and sometimes pointed criticisms and the many instructors in pediatric physical diagnosis at the University of Pennsylvania and Philadelphia General Hospital who gave inestimable aid.

The preparation of the final manuscript would have been impossible without the aid of Drs. Joseph Stokes, Fred Harvie, David Cornfeld, Donald Cornely and David Baker who have generously given of their time and knowledge in correcting the manual. Sections of this manual have been improved with the aid of Dr. Richard Ellis, the Eye; Dr. Philip Marden, Ear, Nose, and Throat; Dr. Joseph Atkins, the Larynx; Dr. Robert Kaye, the Chest; Dr. Sydney Friedman, the Heart; Dr. C. Everett Koop, the Abdomen; Dr. Thomas Gucker, Orthopedics; Dr. Charles Kennedy, the Neurological Examination; and Dr. Albert Kligman, the Skin. Miss L. Plunkett has been most cooperative in preparing many stencils and mimeographs of this material, and its modifications for use by the students, and Mrs. J. White and Miss Lisa Weiss have completed the final typing.

To all these, and to many others whose particular aid cannot at this time be associated with a particular name, I wish to express my sincere thanks. And finally, I should like to thank my wife and daughter for their patience during the many revisions of this manual.

Table of Contents

Introduction

A complete physical examination in a child empha-
sizes many characteristics which differ from those in
adults. It is important to recognize these differences and
also the many variations among normal children.

This is a manual of the special methods used in pediatric physical diagnosis. It is assumed that the person
using it has the basic knowledge of physical examination
of adults, for which many textbooks have been written.
Therefore, no extensive details are listed of the definition
of a sign or of methods of eliciting a sign unless special
methods are used in children. While the material in this
manual includes only the actual physical examination, one
must remember that diagnoses cannot be made by physical
examination alone. Before beginning the examination, it
is important that a careful and detailed history be taken of
the patient and his family, and that this be made part of
the patient's record. As the art of careful observation is
learned, diagnosis by physical examination becomes easier. In the younger child from whom no history can be
directly obtained, or in the child whose parents lack the
ability of accurate observation, this is indeed necessary.

Examples of disease states will be given throughout
the manual. At no time are these states to be considered
the complete differential diagnosis of the sign given. The
examples are given only to present a better understanding
of the sign under discussion. The beginner may use this
manual to learn to elicit a particular sign; the disease
states indicated will later have meaning.

If further examples of a sign are desired, standard
references are suggested. The references used freely in
the development of this manual include the easily available
standard pediatric texts.

There is no "routine" physical examination of a child. Each examination is individualized. Not only are there many physical differences which an examiner accustomed to adults might consider abnormal in a child, but also the variations among a group of children make the examiner more alert to the broad spectrum included in the term "normal." The physician adept at physical diagnosis in children is one who is aware of these variants.

Most of the observed variations can best be explained by the difference in growth rates of the organ systems as they occur from infancy to maturity. For example, the lymphoid tissue is relatively well developed in infancy, becomes maximally developed during childhood, and regresses to small adult proportions at puberty. The nervous system, on the other hand, is largely developed at birth and reaches almost complete adult size by the age of five years. The genital system, however, is infantile until puberty. These and other variations will be noted throughout the discussion of the physical examination.

A question frequently asked by the mother is, "Is my child normal?" One is rarely able at a single observation of that child to tell whether or not he is entirely normal though one may frequently be able to tell that the child is abnormal. Normality in pediatrics, as in statistics, is often confused with the average, and statisticians conclude that there is considerable variation from the average in any normal static population. Normality in children includes the many differences around the average of the age of the child being studied with adequate consideration of the child's background and environment. Determining normality in an ever-changing individual is even more difficult. In conducting a physical examination one looks for normal, variations from normal, and abnormal states. The general mental and physical state, congenital and acquired anomalies, and pathological or disease states are determined.

The record of a complete physical examination in children has special importance not found in that of adults. This record of examination represents a report of one specific time in a child's life when that child is continually and rapidly changing. Therefore, it will be used as a basis for determining whether or not that child is growing and developing normally, according to a group of standards which are learned from books, mothers and patients. More important than a single observation of the child is the use made of this record in following the rate of change of the child at each subsequent examination. The rate of growth, rate of development, and indeed rate of progression of difficulties or anomalies far surpass for evaluation purposes the single examination. The single examination is valuable, of course, not only for determining acute illnesses, but also for determining for the physician, the parent and the child the gross evaluation of the potentialities and liabilities of the child. Thus, even small and apparently insignificant variants should be noted for each child, so that their importance may be adequately assessed in later examination.

For example, if it is known that a particular child with nausea and vomiting was adequately examined two weeks before his illness, that the liver was not palpable at that time, but it is now palpable 2 cm. below the right costal margin, attention would be directed to the liver as a possible cause of the illness. In contrast, if it were known that two weeks before the acute illness the child's liver was palpable, less attention would be paid to the now palpable liver. This type of notation is especially important for so-called "innocent" murmurs of childhood, which are notorious for their frequent change, the significance of which may take many months and many examinations to determine.

The physical examination in a child should also be a record which can be easily interpreted by other physicians. In the appendix, therefore, is included a form for recording a physical examination. Though the method of recording the physical examination is in a logical order, the examination itself is not necessarily performed in this order.

The references used freely in the development of this manual include: Nelson, W. E., Vaughan, V. C., and McKay, R. J.: Textbook of Pediatrics, 9th ed., Philadelphia, W. B. Saunders Company, 1969; Barnett, H. L.: Pediatrics, 14th ed., New York, Appleton-Century-Crofts, Inc., 1968; Green, M., and Richmond, J. B.: Pediatric Diagnosis, Philadelphia, W. B. Saunders Company, 1954; Adams, F. D.: Physical Diagnosis, 13th ed., Baltimore, Williams & Wilkins Company, 1942; Davison, W. C.: The Compleat Pediatrician, 6th ed., Durham, Duke University Press, 1949; and Harvie, F. H.: Pediatric Methods and Standards, Philadelphia, Lea & Febiger, 1962.

CHAPTER I

Approach to the Patient

Every doctor has a series of tricks of examination which he has developed with experience. With an older child cooperation may be improved by such things as flattery of the patient's dress, conversation with the patient on his own level and a discussion of mutual interests. For the preschool child the physician may reassure and distract the patient with interesting objects. Frequently, a two- to four-year-old will remain quiet and apparently interested if the examiner starts a pointless story, particularly about imaginary animals, and asks the patient equally pointless questions about these animals. For the infant one must sometimes resort to various physical measures such as sugar-feeding to keep the patient quiet. Even a two-year-old may respond to flattery and, although bribery of any kind is normally deplorable, a judiciously offered lollipop may create an everlasting attachment between patient and physician.

Usually, the examination is performed while the parent is present. If the child is frightened or clings to the parent, sending the parent out of the room usually serves only to frighten the child more. On rare occasions the parent may be asked to leave the room, but this should be done before the examination begins, or preferably before the doctor enters the room for the examination. Before beginning the examination, one should always wash his hands with warm water. This serves to cleanse and warm the hands so that the patient is not made uncomfortable. The parents also become aware of the consideration of the doctor and appreciate routine hand washing. If the mother stands at the examining table, she should be at the baby's feet. The physician should organize his approach so that a part is examined only once.

In general, one begins a physical examination using no instruments and gradually introduces the various necessary examining equipment. Frequently, a tentative diagnosis can be made simply by observing the child in the mother's arms or as he walks or stands in the room. This diagnosis may then be confirmed following the thorough examination. Usually, the patient is examined in a crib or on a table. The examining table or bed should be large enough so that the child will have no fear of falling, and high enough so that the doctor can examine the patient in comfort.

Physical examinations are performed in children by taking full advantage of opportunities as they present themselves. Anyone concerned with the physical and mental habits of children realizes that he must use all the wiles at his command to establish rapport with the child. The order of an adequate examination, therefore, is more or less determined by the child rather than the physician.

The examination is usually performed with the patient in the position most suitable to him. An infant or severely ill child, or a child who understands well, may be conveniently examined largely in the supine position. However, a six-month-old may have just learned to sit up and may be anxious to demonstrate this ability. Therefore, the examination should be done chiefly with the patient in the sitting position. Likewise, some children may prefer being examined while standing or in unusual positions, and these preferences should be respected if they will not interfere with a complete examination. It is especially important that the child with respiratory distress be examined in the position of most comfort and to provide the best airway, usually in a sitting or sometimes prone position.

An obstreperous or frightened patient, however, may reject all attempts at examination, but frequently even he can be examined completely in his mother's arms. This is especially the position of preference for many one- to three-year-olds. Other children may have such parts as their ears or mouth examined while being held by the mother (Fig. 1). If the patient clings to his mother, his

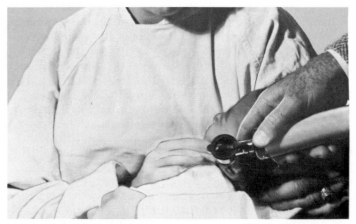

Fig. 1. The child is restrained in the mother's arms and the ears are examined.

back and extremities may be examined in this position and the remainder of the examination can be done later with the patient on his back. It is usually unsatisfactory to attempt to examine the abdomen of a child in his mother's lap. If the mother is helping to restrain the patient she should be told to hold the patient's hands rather than arms. If she holds the arms, the hands are free to interfere with the examiner.

Occasionally, it may be necessary to restrain the patient for the examination of such parts as the ears or mouth. This may be done by placing the infant's arms under his back so that his own weight rests on his palms. The head may be restrained by either examiner or mother and the examination proceeds. An alternate method of restraint is "mummifying" the infant (Fig. 2). His right arm is wrapped with a fold of a sheet. Both ends of the sheet are pulled tight under his back and the left arm is wrapped with the doubled sheet which is then brought back and tucked under the patient's back. The head is restrained as before.

Most pediatricians, aware that the sight of many instruments may frighten the child, start the physical ex-

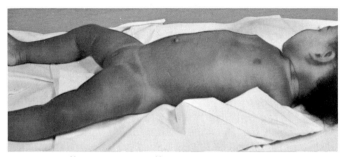

Fig. 2. "Mummifying" the patient. Sheet is drawn
under body and around both arms.

amination with observation of the hands and feet, then
chest or abdomen; then auscultate, percuss, and palpate
these areas, and follow with the remainder of the examination. The genitalia, femoral areas, and anus can be
examined next in boys and younger girls, but these areas
are examined last in older girls. Next, it is usually convenient to examine the head, eyes, face and neck, then
the ears, nose, and throat. In the older girl the labia and
introitus are then examined. Blood pressure, measurements, and testing of the mass reflexes then conclude the
examination in the younger child. In the older child blood
pressure and other measurements are determined first,
and then the examination may proceed from the head downward systematically as in the adult. While performing the
examination it often helps if the examiner allows the patient to play with the instruments he is going to use or has
just finished using. When cooperation is desired for the
more difficult procedures, the patient should be told
firmly what he is to do, rather than be asked to do something.

Before anything frightening or painful is contem-
plated, the patient should be told what is to be done and
what is expected of him. Such procedures as examination
of the head, where the instruments are stuck into the ears
and mouth, or the rectal examination, should be reserved
for the end of the examination. Rectal examination is done

whenever the patient has any symptom referable to the gastrointestinal tract. If the child is old enough to understand, he should be told that these procedures are "uncomfortable but not painful."

Any discomfort caused a patient should be for as short a time as possible. If the doctor feels that at any time in the examination he must hurt the patient, the patient should not be told otherwise during the entire visit. Of course, if the child is acutely ill or hyperirritable, one takes little time for the amenities and proceeds rapidly with the examination.

Occasionally, especially in the acutely ill patient, the physician may have suspicions regarding a particular diagnosis and may wish to confirm or eliminate this diagnosis before proceeding with the examination. For example, if meningitis is suspected in an infant, the fontanel may be palpated first; or if acute abdomen or congenital heart disease is suspected, the abdomen or heart might be examined first. Caution in following such a procedure is necessary. Too frequently, a relatively unimportant secondary diagnosis may be found and the examiner may forget to complete the examination which would reveal the primary diagnosis.

Caution must also be observed in following this procedure in those children with obvious skin blemishes or other gross deformities or in those with suspected psychiatric difficulties or mental deficiency. In these children it is especially desirable to examine first those areas in which difficulty is not expected in order to avoid drawing the attention of the child or the parent to the obvious difficulty.

Ordinarily, the complete physical examination should take the experienced physician no longer than five to ten minutes to perform. Speed is necessary to avoid exhausting the patient. At each visit, regardless of the chief complaint or reason for the visit, a complete systematic examination should be performed and any abnormalities recorded. It is a striking fact that few doctors miss diagnoses because of ignorance; errors are caused by careless omission of simple procedures.

During each examination the child should be completely undressed so that the entire body may be examined. If the room is cool or if the patient is modest or frightened, first one group of clothes may be removed and replaced, and then another. Degree of modesty varies greatly among children. Modesty should be respected in a child regardless of age.

Above all, the successful doctor caring for children must obtain genuine pleasure from examining and dealing with them. He should be friendly and unharried, and he must proceed with the examination with interest, patience, dexterity and confidence.

CHAPTER II

Measurements

The usual measurements taken at a physical examination include temperature, pulse rate, respiratory rate,
height, weight and blood pressure. For the child under
two years of age circumference of head, chest and abdomen are noted. These measurements are ordinarily taken
at the very end of the examination but are recorded first.
Other measurements, such as chest and pelvic width,
crown-rump, and sitting and standing height are ordinarily
not determined in the physical examination except as indicated.

TEMPERATURE

The temperature is best taken either immediately before starting the physical examination or after it is over.
Temperatures are probably of more value to the parents
than to the physician. If a patient is ill, one degree more
or less of fever does not mean one degree more or less of
disease. However, parents like to know how many degrees
of fever their children have and they can be reassured if
the temperature is found to be normal.

A satisfactory routine temperature can be obtained
in children under six years of age by placing the thermometer in the axilla or groin, putting the arm or the leg along
the patient's body, and holding the arm or leg against the
thermometer for three minutes. In general, axillary or
groin temperatures are about two degrees lower than rectal or one degree lower than oral temperatures.

If a rectal temperature is desired, the thermometer
is well greased and is inserted past the mercury bulb. The
child is placed face down across the mother's lap with the

legs dangling alongside the mother's leg. The mother
holds the buttocks firmly with one hand and the arm of
that hand lies firmly across the child's back. The thermometer is inserted about 1 inch and held with the other
hand. The thermometer should be held by the parent or
physician as long as it is in place. One should not attempt
to take the rectal temperature in children with rectal diseases or vulvovaginitis. Rectal temperatures are more
frequently elevated than oral temperatures following exercise. Rectal temperatures should never be taken with
the child lying on his back, as the thermometer will then
be inserted at the wrong angle, increasing chances of
breaking the thermometer or perforating the rectum.

The oral temperatures should not be taken until the child
understands well what is expected of him, usually beyond
six years of age. The newer electronic thermometers
are rapid and accurate and can be used in any orifice at
any age.

The newborn child may have an axillary temperature
of 92 to 97 F., and only after one week is it stabilized at
97 F. axillary.

Fever is a manifestation of increased metabolism
and may be caused by many varied disorders. A body
temperature of 104 to 105 in a child corresponds roughly
in significance to a temperature of 101 to 102 in an adult.
Children may have elevated temperatures normally, after
eating, after vigorous playing, in the afternoon or with
excitement. Children up to six or even eight years of age
frequently get temperature elevations to 104 with minor or
major bacterial, viral or protozoan infections, dehydration or heat stroke. Upper respiratory infections or kidney infections in the infant, or sinusitis, otitis or pro-
dromal stages of the infectious diseases in the older child,
are particular infections which may be difficult to determine on examination but which frequently cause fever.

Fever may also be noted in children with brain injury, particularly cerebral hemorrhage or brain tumor,
in those with maldevelopment of the brain, and in those
who are unable to sweat because of poisoning (especially
atropine) or because of ectodermal dysplasia. Transfu-

sion reactions, intravascular hemolysis or infection and
sickle cell crisis may also be accompanied by fever.
Large daily temperature variations are sometimes noted
with septicemia, liver or kidney disease, tumors, rheumatoid arthritis, Hodgkin's disease or leukemia. Persistent
low grade temperature elevations to 102 F. are seen often
with rheumatic fever and other connective tissue diseases,
but may also be found in a host of other conditions.

Temperature elevations over 104 F. axillary, especially if the rate of elevation is rapid, are sometimes accompanied by convulsions in young children with no other
evidence of convulsive disorders. An elevation of this degree in a child who looks well, is playing and has no obvious disease, may indicate the presence of roseola infantum.

Hypothermia is usually due to chilling but is also seen
in shock states. Especially in infants, however, one frequently notes a normal or low body temperature despite
overwhelming infections.

PULSE

Pulse rate is obtained in young infants either by palpation or by auscultation over the heart, in older children
at the wrist. The significance of the pulse rate, rhythm
and quality will be discussed with the examination of the
heart.

RESPIRATORY RATE

Respiratory rate is obtained by watching, palpating
or auscultating the chest. In young children, accurate
respiratory rates are obtained only during sleep. The significance of the respiratory rate is discussed in the examination of the lungs. However, it is stressed here that
children with a rapid respiratory rate usually have respiratory distress or severe infection, and children with a slow
respiratory rate usually are free from respiratory difficulty.

HEIGHT

Height or length of the child is measured. This measurement, together with weight, is not only a good measure of the over-all growth of the child, but also provides a record of the rate of growth for easy comparison with similar children of similar stature and age as recorded in various standard charts. One of the prime characteristics which distinguish a child from an adult is measurable growth and, if failure of growth is noted, some difficulty in the development of the child should be suspected.

Measurements in the infant are made with the patient flat on his back. The zero end of the tape is held at the infant's heel and the reading at the head is estimated to the nearest half inch. The older child who can stand is measured on the scale. At this time it is valuable to record also the approximate height of both parents and the grandparents.

Even after broad allowances are made for normal variations and the child still appears abnormal in height, consideration must be given to the variations in time of growth. Some children grow rapidly at one age and more slowly at another and these growth spurts may not correspond to the average. If growth still appears abnormal, other explanations must be sought.

The most usual cause of unusual growth apparently is genetic influence. Though height is not strictly inherited, tall parents tend to have taller children than short parents.

Abnormal shortness related to charts with standard deviations may be due to any chronic disease affecting absorption or utilization of nutrients including malnutrition, psychic disturbances, food allergy, food fads, kidney disease, heart disease, liver disease, pancreatic fibrosis or other types of gastrointestinal disorders or anomalies. Children with mental deficiency, any of the hemolytic anemias, rickets or juvenile diabetes may also be short. Dwarfing may be noted in children with disorders of the pituitary, thyroid, parathyroid, adrenal or sex glands. Dwarfism may also be due to the chondrodystro-

phies or other diseases involving the spine, or no cause
may be found.

It is necessary to compare <u>sitting height</u> with total
height in children suspected of being dwarfs. Sitting
height is most easily determined by sitting the child on a
hard surface with his back against the wall and measuring
from the top of his head to the surface. Normally, sitting
height accounts for approximately 70 per cent of total
height at birth, and decreases to about 60 per cent at two
years and about 52 per cent at 10 years. If the sitting
height is greater than one-half the standing height, the patient is said to have infantile stature; if the sitting height
is approximately one-half the standing height, he has adult
type stature.

The early attainment of adult body proportions occurs in children with sexual precocity, and in dwarfs with
Morquio's disease, gargoylism or progeria. Persistently
infantile stature or the late development of adult body proportions is seen in children with delayed adolescence,
hypothyroidism, and some chondrodystrophies. Small
children with normal body proportions may have genetically
small stature, or may be children with pituitary or pri-
mordial dwarfism, or may have gonadal dysgenesis.

Abnormally <u>large growth</u> is rare and usually follows
overfeeding or overeating, perhaps of psychic origin. It
is also seen in children with mental deficiency. True
gigantism due to excess growth hormone from an over-
active pituitary is very rare.

WEIGHT

A child should be weighed routinely at least once a
month for the first six months of life, once every three
months for the next six months, twice a year for the next
three years and yearly thereafter. The same general con-
siderations of growth and development applied to height
apply also to weight, except that, because weight is a
more accurate and more easily obtainable measurement
than height, it may be a more quickly recognizable index
of abnormality than height. The weight of the child should
be compared with standard height-weight charts and due

allowances made for the wide normal variations. But
again, a single measurement tells little compared to the
information obtained from serial measurements which
tell whether the patient is gaining well, too much or too
little.

Acute weight loss indicates acute illness, dehydration
or malnutrition, and chronic weight loss suggests chronic
disease states. These include improper food or feeding,
diarrhea, pancreatic fibrosis or other gastrointestinal
disturbances, emotional difficulties, respiratory difficulty
during feeding, mental retardation, renal, cardiac or connective tissue diseases, and many others.

Rapid weight gain may indicate overhydration or the
appearance of edema, but usually indicates overfeeding or
overeating. A general overweight state, or true obesity,
is usually due to overfeeding or overeating with a usually
discernible psychological background, but may be due to
decreased activity, mental deficiency or intracranial disorders. Rarely, endocrine disorders such as hyperadre-
nalism or hypothyroidism may be associated with obesity.
In contrast to the obesity of overeating, these disorders
are associated with retardation of linear growth.

HEAD AND CHEST CIRCUMFERENCES

The head and chest circumferences are determined
immediately after the length in the infant under two years
of age. They are ordinarily not obtained in children over
two years of age. The head is measured at its greatest
circumference; the chest circumference is obtained at the
nipple-line. One measurement is of little value without
the other.

At birth the average head circumference is 13-
14-1/2 inches (34-37 cm.), and the chest is about 2 cm.
less. The head is usually about the circumference of the
chest until the child is approximately two years old. After
this age, the chest continues to grow rapidly while the head
circumference increases only slightly. Significance of head
and chest measurements is discussed in Chapter IV.

BLOOD PRESSURE

Blood pressure determinations in children are frequently overlooked, but not for good reason. Forgetfulness or lack of proper equipment is the usual reason given for not obtaining a determination which may lead to the proper diagnosis.

Blood pressure is best obtained either before the examination of the head or after the examination is complete and the child is dressing. Preferably, he should be relaxed and not crying. Usually, one compares the cuff to a balloon before applying it and allows the patient to pump the cuff before it is wrapped. After wrapping the cuff snugly, the manometer is placed so that the patient as well as the doctor can see the "silver streak" of the mercury or the "clock" of the spring manometer. The bell stethoscope is placed over the brachial artery.

The proper cuff size is one which is no less than one-half and no more than two-thirds the length of the upper arm. Similar relative sizes are used for the thigh if leg pressures are taken. A larger cuff is difficult to apply and may give readings which are too low. A smaller cuff gives readings which are too high. The rubber bag inside the cuff must itself be long enough to encircle the arm completely.

If the pulse cannot be auscultated, a rough estimate can be made by applying the cuff in the usual manner, slowly deflating, and palpating the radial, popliteal or dorsalis pedis arteries. The first pulsation felt is about 10 mm. below the true systolic pressure. If these arteries cannot be felt, the hand, wrist and forearm (or toes, ankle and leg) can be elevated and tightly wrapped to exclude blood up to the point where the cuff is applied. The cuff is then inflated to a level above the suspected blood pressure. The wrappings are removed. The pressure in the cuff is slowly reduced and the first flushing noted in the hand or foot is close to the systolic pressure. Alternatively, after applying the cuff, the principle of the Doppler effect can be utilized by a ray of ultrasonic energy beamed from a transducer to a blood vessel. The receptor can use earphones or electronic recorder.

If one fails in the first attempt at obtaining the blood pressure, the cuff should be completely removed before again attempting it, as even a deflated cuff may hurt or frighten the child. If an elevated blood pressure is obtained, the measurement should be repeated and the pressure should be measured in the three other extremities. In any patient suspected of having heart disease, the blood pressure should be obtained in the four extremities.

Blood pressure at birth is about 60-90 systolic and 20-60 mm. diastolic. Both pressures usually rise 2-3 mm. per year of age; adult levels are reached near or shortly after puberty. Crying or apprehension may double these levels. Pulse pressure is normally 20-50 mm. during the whole of childhood. Systolic pressure in the arms may equal that in the legs up to about one year. Thereafter the leg pressure should be about 10 to 30 mm. higher than that of the arms. The diastolic pressure should be almost equal in the arms and legs. If it is not, it is an indication that the cuff size is proper for the arms but too small for the legs. Very large differences in arm and leg systolic pressures are suggestive of aortic insufficiency (Hill's sign).

Elevated blood pressure values, both systolic and diastolic, may be noted especially in children with any renal disease including pyelonephritis, acute or chronic glomerulonephritis, the nephrotic syndrome or, rarely, renal calculi. Elevated blood pressures may also be found in children with increased intracranial pressure, adrenal hyperfunction, vitamin A or D poisoning or connective tissue diseases. Elevated blood pressure may also be found in children with bulbar poliomyelitis, usually during the acute phase of the disease. The mechanism is unknown, but may be due to the loss of a depressor reflex. Spinal cord lesions alone may cause hypertension. An elevated blood pressure is usually found in one or both upper extremities of children with coarctation of the aorta.

Unequal blood pressures in the arms occur in children with the scalenus anticus syndrome with cervical rib, or with a coarctation of the aorta, proximal to the left subclavian artery. Some children with patent ductus arteriosus have unequal arm blood pressures.

Elevated systolic pressure alone, with a broadening of the pulse pressure, is noted after exercise or excitement or in febrile states and is usually seen with a lowered diastolic pressure in children with patent ductus arteriosus, arteriovenous fistula or aortic regurgitation.

Normal or elevated diastolic pressure with a low systolic pressure, and therefore a narrow pulse pressure, is noted in children with aortic or subaortic stenosis. A narrow pulse pressure is noted in children with hypothyroidism, a widened or elevated pulse pressure in children with hyperthyroidism.

Low blood pressures are noted in children with cardiac failure, states of shock due to such various causes as heat exhaustion, circulatory collapse, blood loss and adrenal insufficiency. Low blood pressure due to adrenal insufficiency is seen in the newborn with trauma in the adrenal areas, in children with meningococcemia and occasionally other septicemias and in children with chronic disease states or malnutrition.

Orthostatic hypotension is rarely encountered in children. When found, it is probably due not to pooling of blood in the lower extremities, but rather to some reflex vasodilatation or lack of vasoconstriction on assuming an upright posture.

CHAPTER III

General Appearance, Skin, Lymph Nodes

The general appearance of the child may reveal much more than subtle physical findings. When first seeing a child, it is well worth while to sit down and slowly observe him: Does he look well or ill? Does he appear comfortable or uncomfortable? If uncomfortable, in what way or how does he appear to be uncomfortable? Is he breathing easily or with difficulty? Is he in any type of physical or emotional distress? Is he alert or lethargic? Is he clean or dirty? Is he cooperative or belligerent? Does he have any gross abnormalities or anomalies? Is he fat or thin, tall or short? Does he look malnourished? Is he apprehensive, and, if so, is this due to new surroundings, to his parents, to the examiner or to his disease? Is he interested in the new instruments presented to him? Does he obey his mother and the doctor or does he fight them? If he obeys, is this through fear or is he happy to obey? Is he excited or calm? Does he twitch and fidget? In essence, does he appear to be similar to his peers or different, and if different, how does he differ?

A statement of the general appearance should describe the facies of the child and should tell whether the child appears well or in acute distress, chronically ill, alert, comatose, delirious, lethargic, dull, bright, responsive, hostile, cooperative or by the use of other helpful descriptive terms it should start the examiner off on the road to proper diagnosis. Note is also made of the interaction between the patient and his parents during the entire examination. Pediatricians are fortunate in that their patients, unlike adults, rarely dissimulate. Regardless of what the mother says about the patient, the experienced pediatrician knows that a child who does not look ill is usually not acutely ill and the child who looks ill usually is acutely or chronically ill.

During the course of each examination, the child should be completely undressed. In the infant, this is most easily accomplished by having the mother completely undress the child before the examination. In the older child any shyness should be respected and the patient should be examined piecemeal and covered completely thereafter.

If the patient is acutely ill, one tries to determine the system involved and the degree of distress. For example, flaring nostrils point to the respiratory or cardiac systems and delirium, coma or convulsions to the central nervous system. The nature of the cry of the child should be noted. A strong loud cry may indicate that the child is in pain or is frightened, or may indicate simply that the child wishes to cry. Even a strong cry is helpful in diagnosis in that it usually indicates that the child is not weak or debilitated. A weak cry, on the other hand, may indicate that the child is weak, debilitated, or gravely ill. A screeching, high-pitched cry may indicate that the child has increased intracranial pressure or other central nervous system lesion. A hoarse, low-pitched cry in an infant may be normal or may occur in children with laryngeal abnormalities, tetany, or cretinism.

The facial expression and appearance of the child is known as the facies; it should be noted and described. A normal newborn may be asleep or crying, but all other children are responsive during the examination. The child who is smiling, chattering, and laughing is usually well or only moderately ill. The child who cries constantly may be more seriously ill.

A child who lies quietly with few movements, staring into space, may be gravely ill. The child with paradoxical hyperirritability may lie quietly on the examining table only to scream when picked up by the mother. This is a valuable sign, since most children are calmed when picked up, and may indicate a serious disturbance in the central nervous system, particularly meningitis, or pain in motion such as occurs with scurvy, fracture, cortical hyperostosis, or acrodynia; or it may represent a serious disturbance in response to painful stimuli.

A child with acute illness may have parched skin and tongue, sunken dry eyes, weak cry and an exhausted and lethargic behavior. This appearance also may be seen in children with dehydration or acute or chronic malnutrition. The eyes may appear bright and apprehensive in patients with febrile states.

An appearance which indicates pain is easily recognized, with wincing, crying, doubling up, rubbing the hand over the painful part, general fretfulness and other similar signs of discomfort. The cause of the pain, of course, must be determined. This type of painful facies may be modified in a few disease states. For example, with peritonitis the child lies ominously still, the nares flare and respiration is entirely thoracic and very shallow. With intussusception the child lies very still one moment and the next moment he claws, twists and screams. Watch the face of the child as you examine other parts of the body. Palpation over a tender abdomen elicits a grimace in the stoic as he says "It doesn't hurt." A grimace or changing cry as you palpate over the bladder or in the costovertebral angle may be a real sign of renal disease, previously unsuspected.

The dyspneic child is characterized by very rapid respiration, flaring of the nares and perhaps some cyanosis about the lips. The child may be irritable and hyperactive, perhaps apprehensive, and appear to be fighting for air. With carbon dioxide retention, confusion, stupor and finally shock may be added to these signs.

The facies of a child with nasal obstruction is characterized by mouth breathing, open mouth, narrow pinched nose, high palate, dull appearance, nasal voice and may be accompanied by a sunken sternum. This type of facies may occur in children with choanal nasal atresia, but more commonly it is due to hypertrophied adenoids or chronic sinusitis.

The facies of a mentally deficient child is sometimes diagnostic. The eyes are dull, the face is blank and the child is unresponsive. An excellent characterization of

this is given by James Thurber (Thurber Country, Simon
and Schuster: New York, 1953, p. 37) as his description
of the housewife who has the radio on all day, and which
he describes as the "Network Look": "...an adenoidal
dropping open of the mouth and a vacancy in the eyes, as
if perception had just moved out of the mind." Mental deficiency in children may be due to hereditary factors, maternal infections, especially in the first trimester of pregnancy, congenital anomalies of the brain or degenerative
neurologic disorders; commonly it is due to cerebral injury or sequelae of infections, and it is frequently accompanied by other signs of cerebral palsy. Mental deficiency must not be assumed, however, in all children
with dull expression. Children who are deaf or blind or
who have specific language difficulties and children with
prolonged illness or psychologic difficulties may have a
similar facies, easily mistaken for mental deficiency.

The position the child assumes during the examination should be noted. Abnormal, resistant or persistent
positioning may be due to muscular, neurological or emotional disorders. For example, the child with torticollis
or with cerebellar disease may lean his head toward the
affected side; the child with appendicitis or other painful
intra-abdominal conditions may lie on the affected side
with the leg of that side flexed at the hip and knee; the
child with unilateral labyrinthitis may insist on lying only
on the affected side.

Likewise, voluntary or involuntary movement or
lack of movement may direct attention to a particular system. For example, the brain-injured child with spastic
paresis may keep his arm flexed at the elbow and his wrist
and fingers may be held stiffly in flexion; the brain-injured
child with extensive cerebral involvement may be entirely
in extensor spasticity; with cerebellar involvement, he
may be ataxic; or with basal ganglia involvement, he may
be athetoid and grimacing.

The state of nutrition is estimated. Acute malnutrition manifests itself as loss of weight and skin turgor, discussed later. Chronic malnutrition may be indicated by
poor weight gain, bony prominences, protuberant abdo-

men, flat buttocks, prominent sucking pads in the cheeks, muscle wasting, poor muscle tone and slow response to stimuli.

Overnutrition is recognized as obesity and unusual weight gain. Causes of weight loss and gain have been discussed in the section on Weight.

Development is noted. The physician notes the patient's response to himself and the child's surroundings by speech, action and crying, and makes a rapid estimate of mental development. Gross deviations from the normal can be seen at a glance if the child appears dull or does not respond. Gross physical development for the age is estimated and is confirmed by direct measurement.

Speech is one of the developmental signs least subject to motor difficulty, and should be noted in almost the youngest child. A three-month-old may "coo" and a seven-month-old may say "ma-ma" and "da-da." A few more words are added at one year, and short sentences can be made out at two years. The three-year-old, even if not frightened, may stutter or stammer. Failure to develop speech may be due to motor incoordination of the speech muscles, but is commonly due to a lack of desire to speak due to adequate communication by other means. Such children respond to simple commands readily. Other causes of failure to speak include lack of stimulus by parents or environment, deafness, mental retardation, histidinemia or psychological disturbances.

A convenient record of development can be kept with the Denver Developmental Screening Test (Appendix II).

ODOR

Some infants and children will have distinct body odors. A few of these odors are associated with diseases. A musty or mousy odor is found in children with phenylketonuria or diphtheria. The odor of maple syrup is found in children with maple syrup urine disease; the odor of sweaty feet, in infants with isovaleric or n-butyric/n-hexanoic acidemia. Children smelling like a brewery or like fish may have a defect in methionine metabolism, known as

oasthouse disease.   Acetone odors may occur in children
with any acidosis, particularly diabetic ketoacidosis.

SKIN

While observation of the skin is the sine qua non of
dermatologic diagnosis, palpation of skin lesions should
not be neglected.   The skin may be examined as a whole
or as each underlying part is examined; however, regardless of the method adopted, the condition of the skin of the
entire body should be noted at each examination.   If skin
lesions are found, their distribution, color and character
are noted.

The color of the skin is noted.   Normal pigmentation
is due to melanin in the skin; depigmented areas are termed
"vitiligo."   Vitiligo in small patches in children may be the
first sign of tuberous sclerosis or other neuroectodermal
disease.   Generalized lack of pigmentation occurs in albinism, an inborn error of tyrosine metabolism, and the
Chediak-Higashi syndrome.   Localized areas of increased
pigmentation, or nevi, are common.   Size, color, and
presence of hair should be noted.   Various shades of red
nevi are usually of vascular origin (hemangiomas).   Small
vascular nevi due to capillary dilation with small radiating
vessels may be easily compressed.   Because of their appearance they are called spider nevi or spider angiomas.
A few may be present in normal children if on the arms or
hands or high on the face.   These nevi are larger and more
common on the trunk in cirrhosis or hepatitis.   Yellow,
brown or black nevi are usually local melanin deposits.
Multiple small pigmented spots are termed freckles.

Increased dark pigmentation, especially over the exposed areas, is most frequently due to sun or windburn.
Occasionally, increased pigmentation may be due to hypothyroidism, Addison's disease, hemosiderosis, lupus
erythematosus, argyria, pellagra or other deficiency
states.   A pellagralike, symmetrical browning of the
dorsal aspects of the hands on exposure to sunlight may
be associated with cerebellar ataxia in Hartnup's syndrome,
a metabolic defect.   Photosensitivity is also characteristic
of errors in porphyrin metabolism.

Light brown asymmetrical pigmented areas are seen in children with polyostotic fibrous dysplasia. Darker spots (café-au-lait patches), especially if more than five in children under five years of age, or sometimes fibromas along the course of a nerve, are seen in patients with neurofibromatosis. Large flat black or blue-black areas are seen frequently over the sacrum and buttocks. They are termed "Mongolian spots" and have no pathological significance. Bluish-black soft, verrucous symmetrical areas of the axillae, neck, and knuckles are characteristic of acanthosis nigricans, sometimes associated with malignancies, genetic abnormalities, drug use or endocrine diseases.

Cyanosis and jaundice are looked for and should always be noted. Cyanosis is a bluish discoloration of a normally pink area, and is most easily detected in the nail beds or in the mucous membranes of the mouth. It occurs when a minimum of 5 Gm. per cent of reduced hemoglobin is present, regardless of the total hemoglobin. Thus, cyanosis develops less easily in an anemic child, more easily in a child with polycythemia, and not at all in a child with an anemia with hemoglobin content of less than 5 Gm. per cent. Visible cyanosis, it should be remembered, is not a good estimate of degree of oxygen unsaturation except when the total amount of hemoglobin is between 80 and 100 per cent unsaturated. Lesser degrees of unsaturation may be suspected but can be determined only by suitable laboratory tests.

Cyanosis is usually due to pulmonary disease such as atelectasis, pneumonia or pancreatic fibrosis, or to cyanotic congenital heart disease. The most common causes of cyanotic congenital heart disease are transposition of the great vessels, tetralogy of Fallot, tricuspid atresia, total anomalous venous return, truncus arteriosus, pulmonary atresia, and congestive heart failure. Other causes of cyanosis include obstruction of the respiratory tract, prolonged crying, temper tantrums with breath-holding, convulsive states, cardiac failure, acrocyanosis and shock. Cyanosis is seen with as little as 1-2 Gm. per cent of abnormal hemoglobin due to poisoning as in methemoglobinemia and sulfhemoglobinemia.

The upper and lower extremities are compared with respect to cyanosis. The lower extremities may be more cyanotic than the upper in patients with infantile coarctation·of the aorta and also in patients with pulmonary hypertension with patent ductus arteriosus. The lower extremities may be less cyanotic than the upper in children with transposition of the great vessels with patent ductus.

Veins are normally seen through the thin skin of many children. Distended veins in the arms and legs are usually due to dependent position. Dilated veins elsewhere may be due to cardiac decompensation or local venous obstruction and also are seen in cyanotic children. Collateral arterial circulation is seen rarely in children.

Direction of blood flow should be determined if fistula, collateral circulation or obstruction is suspected. First the vessel is emptied by placing two fingers together and then pushing one finger along the course of the vessel for one or two inches. If the vessel fills before pressure is released, collateral circulation is present. Then, pressure of one finger is released. If the vessel fills after release of pressure, blood flow is in the direction from pressure release toward the area where pressure is still applied. If the vessel does not fill, the first finger is replaced, the second is released and similarly observed to indicate direction of blood flow. If the vessel still does not fill, poor circulation in the area is suggested.

The area over a vein may be tender with infection in the vein—thrombophlebitis. When thrombophlebitis becomes extensive and causes obstruction to blood flow, the veins may become tortuous, dilated and easily palpable. Phlebitis of the deep veins of the legs can be elicited by forcibly flexing the foot and noting pain in the calf (Homan's sign). In children, phlebitis usually results from infection spreading from an area near the vein, or from embolism or thrombosis.

Jaundice can be various shades of yellow or green, and is best seen by looking at the sclerae, the skin or the mucous membranes in daylight; it may be missed entirely in artificial light. It occurs in the newborn when the total serum bilirubin is more than 5 mg. per cent, and it is seen in the older child when the total bilirubin is more than 2 mg. per cent. It is caused by cellular or obstructive liver disease, or hemolysis. Common causes of jaundice, in addition to those seen in the newborn period, include any of the hemolytic anemias, many types of poisons, viral hepatitis, infectious mononucleosis; biliary stenosis, atresia or obstruction; leptospirosis and choledochal cyst. Jaundice may also appear with infections anywhere in the body, especially pneumonia and congenital syphilis. Jaundice is rarely caused by bile duct stones in childhood, though these sometimes appear after repeated episodes of hemolysis.

A pale yellow-orange tint of the skin may be due to carotenemia and is most prominent over the palms, soles and nasolabial folds. Carotenemia is due to excess carotene ingestion but may be an early sign of hypothyroidism. Occasionally it occurs in diabetic children. A peculiar yellowness to the skin unrelated to jaundice is seen in children with severe hemolytic anemias.

Pallor or paleness should be noted. In darkly pigmented children, it is most easily detected in the nail beds, conjunctivae, oral mucosa or tongue, which are normally reddish-pink. Pallor should never be considered an accurate estimate of hemoglobin concentration. It is usually a normal complexion characteristic or a sign of indoor living, but it may indicate anemia, chronic disease, edema or shock. Plethora, due to polycythemia, is usually not easily detected in children.

Erythematous lesions of varying types appearing simultaneously, with peripheral spreading and central clearing, are characteristic of erythema multiforme. If these lesions are 2 to 4 cm. in diameter, painful, tender and feel nodular, especially if they are along the shins, they are erythema nodosum. The lesions may be skin manifestations of such systemic diseases as rheumatic fever, drug reactions, streptococcosis, rheumatoid arthritis, Stevens-Johnson syndrome, tuberculosis, lupus erythematosus, or sarcoid. Erythema nodosum is more common in girls, particularly at puberty, than in boys. Similar single lesions on the hands, feet, knees or buttocks, usually making a raised circle with normal skin inside and outside the erythematous area, may be charac-

teristic of granuloma annulare, a disease which may be
due to sensitivity to penicillin or other agents. Non-tender
erythematous patches on the palms and soles, Janeway's
spots, occur in children with acute bacterial endocarditis.
A fleeting, purplish, erythematous rash lasting a few
minutes to a few hours and recurring at short intervals
may be seen in children with rheumatoid arthritis. Erythema which is <u>annular</u> or circinate, 1 to 2 cm. in diameter, serpiginous, not raised, with erythematous margins
surrounding intact skin over the arms, trunk, and legs
but not on the face is erythema marginatum (annulare). It
is characteristic of rheumatic fever. The rash may change
from hour to hour.

  Localized, painful, hot, erythematous, indurated
areas with raised borders are characteristic of erysipelas.
Erysipelas is usually due to streptococcal infection of the
skin and is accompanied by high fever. Localized, painful,
erythematous, hot, indurated areas but lacking the raised
borders are characteristic of cellulitis. Similar-appearing
lesions, particularly around the face, occur with cold injury
and frostbite — cold panniculitis. Cellulitis is due to infection in the subcutaneous tissues and, in children, may over-
lie areas of osteomyelitis in the bone or thrombophlebitis.
Erythematous lines following the course of the lymphatics
are inflamed superficial lymph vessels, lymphangitis.

  The most common erythematous eruptions, however, are of varying extent and may be due to almost any
type of irritation. In the diaper area, erythema is an
early form of diaper rash, a type of contact dermatitis.
Wind, sun, wool or clothing may cause erythema of the
face or other exposed parts. Many other irritants are
equally culpable. Excoriation of the convex surfaces of
the buttocks is usually due to ammonia dermatitis; the region around the anus usually is excoriated after loose
stools, whereas excoriation around the mucocutaneous
area may be due to congenital syphilis. Excoriation of
opposing surfaces, especially in the creases of the neck
or axillae, is intertrigo, and may be due to moisture with
maceration of the skin with constant irritation. The excoriations are red, scaly, and sharply outlined with
monilia infection.

Diffuse redness of the hands and feet, especially if accompanied by severe pain, suggests the diagnosis of acrodynia, though boric acid poisoning may be similar. Intermittent pallor or cyanosis of the fingers and toes may be an early sign of Raynaud's phenomenon. This condition is usually painless, may be aggravated by cold or emotion, and is due to arteriolar spasm with sympathetic nervous system overactivity. Faint erythematous streaks, especially near sites of infection or injury, indicate lymphangitis. Bright confluent erythema of the cheeks, as if slapped, with a warm non-tender skin which blanches on pressure and fades in one to four days is seen in children with fifth disease — erythema infectiosum.

Discrete non-raised lesions are termed macules. The rapid appearance of many macules is characteristic of the exanthemata: measles, German measles, scarlet fever, roseola infantum and typhoid fever. It is sometimes difficult to distinguish these from drug rashes, especially from those due to penicillin or atropine. Similar eruptions may be seen in children with rickettsial diseases or infectious mononucleosis and other viral diseases, particularly the ECHO and Coxsackie groups. Similar eruptions are seen in fourth disease — Dukes' or mild scarlatina — and in erythema infectiosum. A German measles-like rash may occur about 7-10 days after smallpox vaccination.

Firm skin and subcutaneous elevations with discoloration are papules. Papules may occur with any of the exanthemata, following the macular stage, and may also occur following any condition causing the appearance of macules. Small gray or white papules are seen in sarcoid. Red, circular, non-hemorrhagic areas, 1-2 cm. in diameter, over the chest, thighs or elsewhere, with scratch marks, may be due to ringworm. A large, purplish, maculopapular, scaly, oval area surrounded by smaller, similar lesions is found in pityriasis rosea. Sharply raised red scaly areas over the elbows and knees are characteristic of psoriasis.

Skin elevations containing serous fluid are vesicles or blisters. Larger vesicles are termed "blebs" or "bul-

lae." Vesicular lesions of importance in childhood include
chickenpox, where the lesions appear in crops; herpes
simplex or fever blisters about the mouth; herpes zoster,
associated with pain, along nerve pathways; insect bites
or ivy or other poisons, in exposed areas; and molluscum
contagiosum, umbilicated vesicles usually over the abdomen or knees. Smallpox and rickettsialpox are rare.
Lesions are usually in the same stage, vesicles are umbilicated, and are absent from the axilla in smallpox. Lesions
are itching and in varied stages in chickenpox, and may
cover the body, including the axilla and head. Pain pre-
cedes the appearance of vesicles in herpes zoster in contrast
to the other vesicular diseases. Bullae may occur with
burns. Bullae may occur on the palms and soles in children
with scarlet fever or congenital syphilis; rarely, they occur
following irritation in children with the hereditary disease
epidermolysis bullosa, or in children with the bullous form
of erythema multiforme, or with dermatitis herpetiformis.
Bullae occur commonly in children with sunburn or ivy or
oak poisoning. Small vesicles or bullae are also seen on
areas exposed to sunlight in children with recurrent summer
eruption, hydroa estivale. Bullae or other eruptions may
appear in children exposed to sunlight who have congenital
porphyria. Bullae at birth followed by zebralike pigmentation is characteristic of incontinentia pigmenti, a congenital
malformation of the ectoderm. Bullae of the ends of the
fingers are seen in children with diarrhea who have acro-
dermatitis enteropathica. Tender skin with erythema followed by bullae which may rub off occurs in children with
toxic epidermal necrolysis, a severe disease related to
staphylococcal infection.

Skin elevations containing purulent fluid are pustules.
Pustules are usually due to bacterial infection or skin abscesses. Pustules may also be seen following any of the
states causing vesicles, in the adolescent with acne, or in
the child following poisoning as with iodine. Groups of
pustules due to staphylococci or streptococci are known as
"impetigo." Deeper infections, termed "ecthyma," probably
start as impetigo. Larger abscesses of the hair follicles or
sebaceous glands are furuncles or carbuncles. Small

straight lines or burrows, associated with papules, vesicles or pustules, may be scabies, due to the itch mite. These lesions may appear anywhere on the body of the child, in contrast to the more localized distribution on the hands and groin of the adult, and are usually accompanied by signs of itching.

Necrotic areas of the superficial and deep layers of the skin, skin ulcers, common in adults with vascular insufficiency, are rare in children; they occasionally occur on the legs of children with sickle-cell anemia. Ulceration occurs before the healing stage of smallpox inoculations and it may occur following skin destruction by such agents as burns or trauma or following subcutaneous injection of antigens as a result of hypersensitivity.

Petechiae are small reddish-purple spots in the superficial layers of the skin. They frequently indicate severe systemic disease due to bacterial emboli or vascular damage such as occurs with meningococcemia, rickettsial diseases, other overwhelming systemic infections or bacterial endocarditis; inadequate or defective platelets as in thrombocytopenic or non-thrombocytopenic purpura; or increased capillary permeability as in scurvy or leukemia. More frequently they may be caused by injury or increased capillary pressure as with severe coughing, especially pertussis; by allergies in which the cause is unknown, or by direct trauma. Paler, 0.5 mm., red or pink areas may be petechiae or may be rose spots, characteristic of typhoid fever or other Salmonella infections.

Ecchymoses, which are larger evidences of blood under the skin, usually are due to bruising or other injury, but they may be a sign of increased bleeding tendency as in hemophilia, leukemia or the purpuras.

Localized areas of swelling and scratch marks are characteristic of hives (urticaria, wheals), papular urticaria, insect bites, scabies or ivy and sumac poisoning. Localized small swellings or excrescences without scratch marks may be warts.

Increased sensitivity to skin pressure manifested by wheals or bright red lines is characteristic of dermato-

graphia. This is a common disorder of unknown significance. Especially persistent dermatographia, tache
cerebrale, is a sign of central nervous system irritation
particularly noted in patients with tuberculous meningitis.
Dermatographia is easily produced by lightly scratching
the skin with one's nail, and is most easily noted over the
back or upper chest. Large wheal formation after stroking
may be a sign of generalized mast cell disease, urticaria
pigmentosa.

Subcutaneous nodules may be found occasionally.
Usually, they are due to absorbing or calcifying hema-
tomas, to sterile abscesses or to poorly absorbed injec-
tions. Nodules over the extensor surfaces of the joints or
near the occipital protuberances may aid in the diagnosis
of rheumatic fever, especially with severe carditis, or
with rheumatoid arthritis, lupus erythematosus or granuloma annulare. They may be tender. Red, tender nodules
on the finger tips, thumbs or footpads (Osler's nodes) are
pathognomonic of subacute bacterial endocarditis. Absence
of small saucer-like areas of subcutaneous tissue with
button-like nodules under the skin may be due to fat necrosis. Small yellow or orange plaques, xanthomas, may be
seen on the skin, particularly about the nasal bridge. They
are usually due to local accumulations of fatty substance.
Xanthomas may occur as isolated findings, particularly
in infancy, or may be a manifestation of any condition
causing hyperlipemia or of the reticuloendothelioses.
Pigmented or depigmented xanthoma-like lesions may be
adenoma sebaceum, characteristic of tuberous sclerosis.
Cysts may be felt under the skin as superficial masses
with fluid. They are usually non-tender and may transilluminate light. A cyst over the dorsum of the hand or
wrist is most commonly a ganglion, a degenerated cyst of
the tendon sheath. Tumors of the skin may be seen or felt.
These may be firm or soft and are usually lipomas or fibromas. Atrophic areas of the skin may follow injury or
the use of insulin by the diabetic.

Feeling the skin for texture may reveal roughness,
as seen in children commonly during the winter, especially after contact with wool or soap. It may occur in
children with hyperkeratosis due to vitamin A deficiency,

hypothyroidism and hypoparathyroidism. Rough dry skin, especially over the legs, may be a manifestation of ichthyosis. Thickening of the skin in the flexor folds of the elbows and knees is characteristic of chronic eczema. Hardening and thickening of the skin also occurs in sclerema, scleredema, scleroderma and dermatomyositis.

Scaling of the skin is noted. Yellow, dirty scaling beginning on the scalp is termed "cradle cap." Scaling beginning on the scalp and proceeding down the face and body, associated with erythema, is a self-limited form of exfoliative seborrheic dermatitis (Leiner's disease) which appears in the first three months of life. Scaling which begins on the cheeks, spreads to the forehead, scalp, posterior of the ears, and down the body, beginning about the second month of life and lasting one to two years, is characteristic of infantile eczema. Scaling in the diaper area, sometimes associated with vesiculation and infection, may occur with diaper rash, a form of contact dermatitis. Scaling may occur on almost any area of the body at any age due to contact with a large number of agents (contact dermatitis). Scaling between the toes, on the feet or between the fingers may be due to ringworm, epidermophytosis or irritants in the shoes or socks. Scaling, especially of the palms and soles, may occur after any erythematous eruption, particularly scarlet fever, or in infants with congenital syphilis.

Subcutaneous emphysema is felt as a crackling or crepitant sensation under the skin. It is most commonly associated with pneumothorax, pneumomediastinum and gas gangrene. A similar sensation is obtained if an area over a bone fracture is palpated.

Striae are usually pale white or pink lines which occur in localized areas that are growing rapidly, such as the lower abdomen or thighs of an obese child. They usually occur following overeating or during the growth spurt, but striking purple striae may indicate the presence of Cushing's syndrome. Scars are red or white lines and are evidence of previous injury or operation. They are elevated when there is keloid formation.

The degree of sweating is estimated. Infants normally begin to sweat after the first month of age. Sweating, especially in the child under one year of age, may be profuse and is usually due to exercise, crying, an overly warm atmosphere or eating. Profuse sweating in the infant, however, may occasionally be due to fever, hypoglycemia, hyperthyroidism, congenital heart disease, hypocalcemia, acrodynia, pneumothorax, pancreatic fibrosis or fear. A <u>dry</u> skin, anhidrosis, also is normal, but it may be a sign of dehydration, coma, atropine poisoning, hypothyroidism, eczema or ectodermal dysplasia.

The skin is felt for tissue <u>turgor</u> and <u>edema</u>. Tissue turgor is best determined by grasping between the thumb and index finger one or two inches of the patient's skin and subcutaneous tissues over the abdominal wall, squeezing, and allowing the skin to fall back into place (Fig. 3). It is one of the best estimates of status of hydration and nutrition. Normally, the skin appears smooth and firm and, when grasped as described, quickly falls back into place without residual marks. The skin remains suspended and creased for a few seconds in children with poor turgor.

Fig. 3. Subcutaneous turgor. Best demonstrated by grasping the skin and subcutaneous tissue over the abdomen, and allowing to fall back into place.

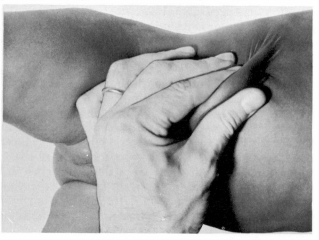

The tissues feel plastic and doughy in children with chronic wasting disease, peritonitis, or hyperelectrolytemia with dehydration. Little subcutaneous tissue will be felt in malnourished children. The skin will remain suspended and in folds in dehydrated patients. This may not occur in obese infants. If dehydration is suspected in them, other signs should be sought. Poor tissue turgor may be apparent in a normal infant a few days old, especially in a premature infant, but he rapidly adds fat and subcutaneous tissue so that turgor is normal by a month of age. The skin, especially over the legs, normally feels firm. It feels thin and loosely filled in children with chronic diseases, malnutrition, and rickets. It may feel very soft and flabby in children with flaccid paralyses and in children with muscle diseases such as myasthenia gravis or amyotonia congenita, as well as in some mental defectives. It may be soft and mushy in mongolism. It may feel hard and thickened in children with hypothyroidism, whether congenital or acquired. Other unusual texture is described in Chapter IX under hardness of the skin, sclerema, and scleroderma.

The skin may be tender to touch. This may indicate that the child is irritable, that he has central nervous system disease, or that he has other systemic illness. It is also tender in children with skin infections or underlying bone or joint infections, or in children with referred pain, particularly from intra-abdominal disease. Skin tenderness is also noted in polyneuritis and over the left shoulder in children with ruptured spleen.

Impressions in the skin which remain for several seconds following finger pressure occur in patients with pitting edema. Edema is the presence of an abnormal amount of extracellular fluid and is caused by an increase of hydrostatic pressure, increased capillary permeability, decreased oncotic pressure, increased retention of sodium or other electrolytes, mechanical obstruction of the lymphatic channels, or decreased excretion of water. Puffy-appearing areas on the body which do not pit or leave marks after pressure or pinching are termed "non-pitting edema." For example, puffy skin without pitting is noted in the cretin.

Edema localized in the eyelids may be the first sign of generalized edema. True, generalized, pitting edema is found earliest over the dependent parts, especially the sacrum and ankles. It is seen in children with kidney disease, malnutrition, especially protein deficiency, terminal liver disease, heart failure of long duration, in adolescent girls before or during the menses, and occasionally without apparent cause over the shins in warm summer weather. It is also seen in children receiving adrenal hormones and in children with hyperaldosteronism or hyperthyroidism.

Localized edema in the eyelids, face or lips may be due to allergy (angioneurotic edema), trichiniasis (trichinosis) or insect bites in those areas. Puffiness of the eyelids may also be seen in children after a long sleep or after crying, and in children with conjunctivitis, frontal or ethmoid sinusitis or cavernous sinus thrombosis. Localized edema of the face may occur following severe cough, as in whooping cough or diphtheria. Facial edema occurs also with mass lesions in the chest, including lymph nodes, as in infectious mononucleosis, which obstruct venous or lymphatic drainage. Edema of the face and eyelids is also common in children with any of the common contagious diseases.

The ridges formed by the raised apertures of the sweat glands make up dermatoglyphics. These are best seen with adequate light and magnification, or by making finger and hand prints. The otoscope without earpiece usually is adequate for both light and magnification. The ridges form arches, loops and whorls on the fingers; where three lines meet, these are triradii. The normal usually has a triradius low on the palm, a triradius with an acute angle in the hypothenar area proximal to the midpalm, and an assortment of arches, loops, and whorls on the finger tips (Fig. 4). Usually, approximately seven or eight finger tips will have ulnar loops and one to three whorls. One arch is not uncommon in the normal. Radial loops are rare in the normal. Deviations from these patterns of seven to eight ulnar loops, one to three whorls, and one or no arch suggest the presence of chromosomal abnormalities, early intrauterine infections, gross abnor-

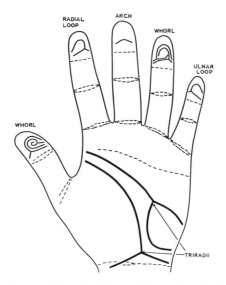

Fig. 4. Normal hand ridges (dermatoglyphics).

malities of growth of the extremities, or some form of
congenital heart disease. A triradius distal to the midpalm
with an obtuse angle is suggestive of Down's syndrome;
arches on all digits suggest trisomy 18. Radial loops may
occur more commonly in children with XXY anomaly, and
large, deep ridges in gonadal dysgenesis. Arches on the
thumbs are common in children with trisomy 15.

NAILS

The nails may be especially valuable areas for determining special disease states. The nail beds are usually the simplest place for determining cyanosis, pallor
or capillary pulsations. Vernix in the newborn can usually be found under the nails. Pitting of the nails is seen
with fungal diseases of the nails and with psoriasis. Yellow staining of the nails is found in the postmature infant.
Darkening of the nails may be noted in children with porphyria. Nails may be absent in children with ectodermal

dysplasia. Infections around the nails, paronychia, are common in children, especially after desquamating skin lesions. They may be bacterial or fungal infections. Hemorrhage under the nails is usually due to injury, or to subacute bacterial endocarditis or the other diseases in which petechiae are noted. The nail beds are characteristically broader than long in children with mongolism, pseudohypoparathyroidism or as a congenital malformation in those syndromes characterized by broad fingers. Spoon-shaped nails with loss of the longitudinal convexity, koilonychia, may be due to fungal infections, iron-deficiency anemia or intestinal diseases, or may be congenital.

HAIR

Hair, other than that of the head, is noted at this time. Hair is sometimes seen over the shoulders and back of newborn, especially premature, infants, but it disappears at about three months of age. Children then do not usually have hair except for scalp, eyebrows and eyelashes, until near puberty. Long eyebrows and eyelashes usually are familial but occasionally appear in children with chronic or wasting diseases.

Unusual hairiness elsewhere on the body, especially over the arms and legs, may be a normal variant or familial characteristic but may be found in children with hypothyroidism, vitamin A poisoning, chronic infections, dilantin sensitivity, or hepatic porphyria. Hairiness of the trunk is noted in children with Cushing's syndrome.

Tufts of hair anywhere over the spine and especially over the sacrum may have special significance. Though resembling a nevus, the hair may mark the site of a spina bifida occulta or spina bifida.

Pubic hair begins to appear at 8 to 12 years of age, followed by axillary hair about six months later and, in boys, facial hair about six months still later. Appearance of hair in these areas indicates normal adrenal and testicular function. Decrease of hair in these areas may be due to hypothyroidism, hypopituitarism, gonadal deficiency or Addison's disease. Early appearance or in-

crease of hair in these areas may be normal, but it may
suggest stilbestrol, testosterone or adrenal hormone ingestion, adrenal hyperplasia or tumor, central nervous
system lesions, pineal hamartoma in boys, polyostotic
fibrous dysplasia, or testicular or ovarian tumors.
Pigmented, coarse, curly or crinkled pubic hair indicates
increased hormonal production and is believed to indicate
onset of sperm formation in boys.

LYMPH NODES

Lymph nodes are generally examined during the examination of the part of the body in which they are located.
These nodes should be routinely palpated: occipital, post-
auricular, anterior and posterior cervical, parotid, submaxillary, sublingual, axillary, epitrochlear and inguinal.
Size, mobility, tenderness and heat are noted. Ordinarily,
shotty, discrete, movable, cool, non-tender nodes up to
3 mm. in diameter are normal in all these areas and, in
the cervical and inguinal regions, nodes up to 1 cm. in
diameter are normal up to the age of 12 years.

Absence of lymph nodes occurs in patients with
agammaglobulinemia.

Large, warm, tender nodes usually indicate acute
infection. Local adenopathy usually indicates local infection but may be a sign of generalized disease.

Generalized adenopathy is seen with such systemic
diseases as bacteremia, streptococcosis, salmonellosis,
syphilis, eczema, infectious mononucleosis, viral hepatitis and measles. Generalized adenopathy, with or without tenderness, may be seen in children with leukemia,
serum sickness, rheumatoid arthritis, lymphomatosis,
Hodgkin's disease or the reticuloendothelial diseases.

A few isolated enlarged nodes may have special significance. Occipital or posterior auricular adenopathy is
seen with local scalp infections, external otitis, German
measles, pediculosis, varicella and tick bite, and with
excessive scratching. The preauricular nodes may be
enlarged with conjunctivitis (Parinaud's syndrome), styes
or chalazion. The "sentinel" node located near the left

clavicle may be the first node enlarged in Hodgkin's disease in children; in adults, this nodal enlargement may indicate gastric cancer. Cervical adenopathy usually accompanies acute infections in or around the mouth or throat, but cool, large, non-tender, matted, cervical glands which may suppurate, especially if unilateral, may indicate tuberculosis. Where adenopathy occurs near a scratch or bite, cat-scratch or rat-bite fever or tularemia is suggested, as well as disease resulting from tick, flea or mite bites or local sepsis. The epitrochlear nodes, in particular, are enlarged in congenital syphilis and cat-scratch disease.

CHAPTER IV

Head and Neck

HEAD

The head is usually held dorsally when the infant is in a prone position by the age of one month. At three months, the normal infant holds his head steady when he is held upright. Failure to hold his head up usually indicates poor motor development. Head nodding may be normal, but it is usually seen in children who are emotionally unstable or mentally retarded or who have spasmus nutans.

Amount, color and texture of the hair is noted. The newborn infant usually has hair which is fully replaced beginning at about three months of age. Lack of hair, alopecia, may be a familial characteristic, a manifestation of ectodermal dysplasia, hyperthyroidism, or progeria. Localized alopecia is seen with ringworm of the scalp, other infections of the scalp and acrodynia; but most commonly, in small infants, it is due to rubbing of localized areas when the infant lies in one position for a long time. Rarely, localized alopecia, alopecia areata, is seen in children with localized syphilis or hypervitaminosis A, in neurotic children who pull out the hair, or following severe systemic disease, e. g. , typhoid fever, collagen diseases such as scleroderma, scalp infections, x-ray, caustics, neoplasms such as lymphoma, carcinoma, mycosis fungoides, after antimetabolites or heparin, or with thallium or arsenic.

Hair normally is smooth with a fine texture. Brittle hair is seen in children with hypothyroidism, hypoparathyroidism, ringworm of the scalp, or arginosuccinicaciduria, a rare inborn error. Fine hair may be seen in any of the states causing alopecia. Fine hair distinguishes the hypothyroidism of hypopituitarism from that of pri-

mary thyroid disease, in which the hair is coarse and
brittle. Twisted, irregularly constricted, woolly or irregularly pigmented hair may each be inherited as an isolated
anomaly. The hair should be examined for the presence
of pediculi or nits.

The shape of the head and face is noted. Marked
asymmetry of the head is found in children with premature and irregular closure of the sutures. Flattening of
part of the head or face occurs in an infant who lies in
only one position or who has unusually soft bones. Thus,
in a child with delayed physical or mental development,
or with rickets, the back of the head will be flat. One
side of the head and face is also flattened in children with
torticollis, or may appear flattened in children with facial
palsy.

The scalp is examined. Special lesions may be noted
in the newborn. Scaling and crusting of the scalp, if generalized, are usually due to seborrheic dermatitis or eczema; if localized, to ringworm of the scalp. Infections
of the scalp, which occur frequently, are noted. Lymph
nodes and subcutaneous nodules are identified by careful
palpation, especially around the occiput.

The sutures are palpated. Usually, they are felt as
ridges until about six months of age. Abnormal sutures,
fractures and fontanels are noted. The posterior fontanel
closes by the second month, the anterior fontanel usually
by the end of the second year. A diagram of the top of the
head, showing the position of fontanels and palpable structures, is shown in Figure 5.

The size and shape of the anterior fontanel are noted
by pressing lightly in the area of the opening. A large
fontanel, over 4 or 5 cm. in diameter, is found occasionally in normal infants under six months of age, but may
also be diagnostic of chronically increased intracranial
pressure, subdural hematoma, rickets, hypothyroidism
or osteogenesis imperfecta.

A tenseness or bulging of the fontanel is best noted
if the patient is in the sitting position. The normal fontanel may feel questionably tense in the infant who is supine. Tenseness may be noted in the crying child but only

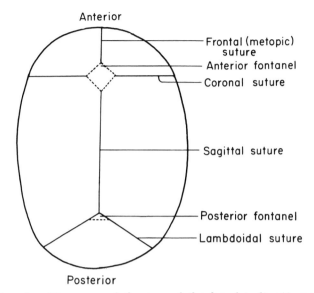

Fig. 5. Diagram of the top of the head indicating position of fontanels and palpable sutures.

during expiration; this physiological bulging disappears when the patient relaxes or inspires. Persistent or true bulging or tenseness of the fontanel is noted in the quiet infant in the sitting position and usually accompanies acute increase in intracranial pressure such as occurs with subdural hematoma, lead poisoning, vitamin A poisoning, brain tumor, sinus thrombosis, cardiac failure, meningitis or encephalitis. Transient bulging of the fontanel has been described in children receiving chlortetracycline, in children with pulmonary diseases, and occasionally in children with roseola and those receiving nalidixic acid.

A depressed fontanel is found with dehydration and malnutrition. A small fontanel is usually normal but it is also an important sign of microcephaly in infants. Occasionally the fontanel is closed with fibrous tissue alone and will feel not quite as firm as the surrounding skull. Fibrous closure should be noted, but physiologically it is

comparable to an open fontanel. Bony closure usually occurs one to two months after fibrous closure. Delayed
closure of the fontanel may occur in children with hydrocephalus, rickets or cretinism. Rarely, delayed closure
is due to syphilis or the osteochondrodystrophies.

Slight pulsations of the anterior fontanel occur in
normal infants. Marked pulsations, however, may be a
sign of increased intracranial pressure, venous sinus
thrombosis, obstruction of the venous return from the head,
or increased pulse pressure due to an arteriovenous shunt,
patent ductus arteriosus or excitement. Aortic regurgitation is a rare cause of increased pulse pressure during the
age when the fontanel is open.

The circumference of the head is measured as described. Until the child is two years of age, the circumference of the head is approximately the same as or slightly larger than that of the chest. Marked disproportions
between the head and chest measurements indicate micro-
or hydrocephaly or increased intracranial pressure. If
the measurements are disproportionate, head and chest
measurements should always be compared with standards,
as the chest itself may be large or small.

Microcephaly may be due to cerebral dysgenesis
alone or to premature closure of the sutures (craniostenosis). Rarely, microcephaly is seen in children with
over-all growth failure.

Hydrocephalus, caused by chronic increase in intracranial pressure, is found by noting the enlarged head, enlarged fontanels, supra-orbital bulging and open sutures.
Dilated scalp veins are characteristic of early hydrocephalus. Hydrocephalus is an enlargement of the ventricular systems of the brain, and may be due to blocking
of the ventricular foramina (non-communicating), blocking of the subarachnoid pathways (communicating), or
rarely failure of the subarachnoid system to absorb
cerebrospinal fluid (external). Hydrocephalus ordinarily
is apparent at birth or shortly thereafter, and is frequently found in children with spina bifida with meningomyelocele. Hydrocephalus starting after birth may be
due to a meningeal infection. That appearing at 4 - 9
months may be due to congenital syphilis.

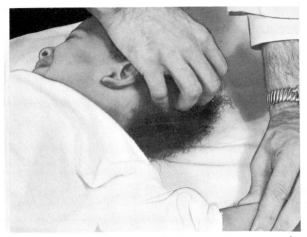

Fig. 6. Position of hand and fingers (examiner's right hand) to palpate for craniotabes.

Bulging of an area of the head occasionally occurs with brain tumors, lacunar defects of the skull and intracranial masses. Bulging of the frontal areas, or "bossing," is characteristic of prematurity, of rickets, and occasionally of congenital syphilis.

Craniotabes is best found by pressing the scalp firmly just behind and above the ears in the temporo-parietal or parieto-occipital region (Fig. 6). The elicitation of a ping-pong ball snapping sensation then indicates craniotabes. It represents a softening of the outer table of the skull. Though the infant sometimes cries, no danger is involved if the pressure is not so excessive that the inner table is pressed. Craniotabes is found in premature infants, in some normal children under six months of age, in babies who lie constantly on one side of the head, and in children with rickets, syphilis, hypervitaminosis A and hydrocephalus.

Macewen's sign is one which many examiners like to elicit, but usually it has little significance in childhood. On percussing the skull with one finger, a resonant "cracked-pot" sound is heard. As long as the fontanel is open, this type of sound is physiological. After closure of the fontanel, the sound indicates increased intracranial pressure or a dilated ventricle.

The head should be percussed in children with neurological disorders in the indirect manner similar to that described for the percussion of the heart. When the head is carefully percussed, one can occasionally elicit dullness near the sagittal sinus. This is a good sign of subdural hematoma.

Tenderness or pain over the occiput may indicate the presence of brain tumor or abscess. Pain over the scalp may accompany cerebral hemorrhage, migraine, trauma, hypertension, vascular neuralgia or anxiety or depressive states. Press hard over the malar bones for a few seconds and then release. Functional headaches may be improved by this maneuver, but headaches with other causes will not change.

In children over two or three years of age the frontal and maxillary sinuses should be percussed in the same manner or by the direct method, for tenderness. Tenderness indicates acute sinusitis. Pressure deep in the bony angle above the inner canthus of the eye frequently elicits tenderness or slight swelling characteristic of acute ethmoiditis. It is difficult and generally unnecessary to transilluminate the sinuses in young children. After the second year, the maxillary sinuses are aerated, and after the seventh year, the frontals can be visualized.

Auscultation over the skull with the bell stethoscope may reveal a swishing sound, bruit, of blood flowing through dilated vascular channels. Systolic or continuous bruits may be heard normally in children up to four years of age or in children with anemia; after this age they suggest the presence of vascular anomalies, especially arteriovenous aneurysms, or increased intracranial pressure. Sometimes similar noise is heard in children with meningitis. Transmitted cardiac murmurs may sometimes be heard as bruits over the skull.

Direction of blood flow in the scalp veins should be determined in children with suspected intracranial abnormalities. It may be necessary first to shave the scalp to determine blood flow, but this procedure occasionally re-

veals abnormal vascularity or vascular channels indicative
of underlying abnormalities. Small ossification defects
may occur in the skull, through which the dura protrudes.
Small defects are termed lückenschädel, and large defects,
encephaloides. Nervous tissue protrudes in children with
encephaloceles. Encephaloceles may be present anywhere
in the skull and are sometimes seen near the inner canthus
of the eye. On the shaved scalp one should note also the
presence of dimples, which may be an indication of a
dermal sinus, or hemangiomas. These are infrequent but
sometimes remediable causes of seizures or meningitis.
Scalp veins may appear dilated in the very young; they
also may indicate the presence of hydrocephalus, tumors,
subdural hematoma, or congenital vascular anomaly.

The skull should be transilluminated in children suspected of having intracranial lesions. A flashlight is fitted
with a piece of sponge rubber so that a tight fit is made
with the scalp. The room must be quite dark. A sharply
delineated area of increased light transmission may be
noted over a subdural hygroma. A bright light should be
placed at the occiput in infants suspected of having anencephaly. In anencephalies, the light will be seen to be
transmitted through the eyes, which the examiner can observe as pinkness of the retina by looking directly into
the eyes.

FACE

Shape of the face is ordinarily noted at the time one
observes the shape of the head. Additional factors other
than those already noted may change the shape of the face.

An easy way to determine facial paralysis is to observe the child while he cries, whistles or smiles. The
paralyzed or weakened side will remain immobile while
the innervated side wrinkles. The lips will rise only on
the intact side, and on the paralyzed side the angle of the
mouth may droop. Wrinkling of the forehead should be
noted.

Unilateral paralysis of the face excluding the muscles of the forehead indicates a central facial nerve (supranuclear) weakness and may be seen in children with cere-

bral palsy or other brain lesions. Unilateral paralysis of
the face including the muscles of the forehead and eyelid
indicates a peripheral facial nerve lesion and may be due
to trauma, otitis media, or other peripheral lesions. Re-
covery from the peripheral facial nerve palsy may occur
in the upper portion of the face first, and at this time may
resemble a supranuclear weakness. Salivary flow can be
measured by putting polyethylene tubes in the submaxillary
ducts. Stimulate salivation by placing a slice of lemon on
the tongue. Count the drops in one minute. Salivary flow,
if measured in a child with peripheral facial palsy, will
be at least 40 per cent of normal in those palsies which
spontaneously recover.

Paralysis and asymmetry about the mouth alone are
usually due to a peripheral trigeminal nerve lesion.

Local swellings about the face are usually due to
edema. Enlargement of the mandibles in infants, however,
may be due to infantile cortical hyperostosis (Caffey's
syndrome) or vitamin A poisoning, and may be mistaken
for parotitis. Large jaws due to fibrous swelling with upward turning of the eyes is seen in cherubism. A small
mandible (micrognathia) is usually a congenital anomaly
but may be seen in children with rheumatoid arthritis.

Local swelling of the parotid glands is best determined by sitting the patient upright, asking him to look
toward the ceiling, and noting the swelling below the angle
of the jaw. Next, run the flat part of the finger downward
from the zygomatic arch. The swollen parotid is then felt.
It is confirmed by allowing the patient to lie on his back.
The parotid then falls back like jelly and pushes the pinna
of the ear forward. Unilateral or bilateral parotid swelling usually is indicative of mumps, but it may be due to a
stone in the parotid duct, allergy, leukemia, or sarcoido-
sis. Parotid swelling with lacrimal duct swelling is
Mikulicz's syndrome. Parotid swelling due to bacterial
infections sometimes occurs in debilitated children. Tumors and cysts occasionally occur in the parotid area in
children. Firm swelling of the parotids, parotid sialad-
enitis, is usually self-limited; it may be caused by animal
scratch diseases, or may be seen in children who com-

pulsively eat starch. Non-tender parotid swelling may
precede the onset of diabetes mellitus.

The area under the jaw is palpated for glands or
tenderness. Submaxillary glands are felt best by palpating
lightly just below the mandible, anterior to the angle of
the jaw, or lightly rubbing this area with the fingertips.
Sublingual glands are similarly palpated just behind the
bony portion of the chin. These glands are ordinarily not
palpable and enlargement or tenderness usually indicates
mumps, cystic fibrosis, local infection or infection in the
teeth or, rarely, stones in the ducts. Unilateral sub-
mandibular or submaxillary swelling is more common
with atypical mycobacteria, bilateral with human tubercle bacilli.

Abnormal or unusual facial appearance is also seen
in many children with generalized dystrophies. Some of
these have characteristic facies, which have been described. Congenital abnormalities may be seen.

Hypertelorism appears to be a large distance between the eyes and occurs with a broadened nasal bridge.
It is measured as an increased interpupillary distance,
and reflects the spacing of the orbits. It is due to over-
development of the lesser wing of the sphenoid bone. If
the medial canthus is displaced lateralward, a similar
appearance may exist. This is called telecanthus. Both
conditions may be normal variants.

Hypertelorism with other mid-facial anomalies
usually occurs in children who are mentally normal. If
hypertelorism is extreme or occurs with anomalies other
than those of the head and face, the probability of mental
retardation is considerable. Infants with hypotelorism
and mid-face anomalies are almost always retarded.
The normal interpupillary space is approximately
3.5-5.5 cm. (Fig. 7).

Twitchings of the face may be seen. These are usually due to tics or habit spasms, but they may be due to
muscular exhaustion or fasciculation.

Chvostek's sign is obtained by tapping the cheek of
the child just below the zygoma with the finger. If the
sign is present, that side of the face will grimace. It is

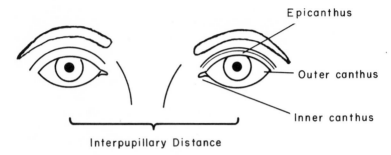

Fig. 7. Measuring interpupillary distance.

difficult to elicit this sign in children under two weeks of
age or in children who are crying. Chvostek's sign may
be present in normal children under one month of age or
over five years of age. In children between these ages,
if this sign is present, it indicates hyperirritability and
may be found with tetanus, tetany or hyperventilation.

EYES

A baby's eyes—
Their glance might cast out pain and sin,
Their speech make dumb the wise
By mute glad God-head felt within
A baby's eyes.   (Source unknown)

     The eye is not only the most important sensory organ,
but also a key to the area behind. A careful examination
of the eye of a small child is done practically without the
cooperation of the child and is difficult. The infant under
one year may be kept quiet with a bottle, but from one to
four years other wiles must be used.
     Even for a small child, the best examination is done
if the examiner makes careful use of his left hand. The
right hand should hold the ophthalmoscope and the left hand
should be far from the patient's eye to attract his gaze.
The natural tendency is to try to hold the eye open forcibly.
This only makes for a wet eye which is impossible to hold

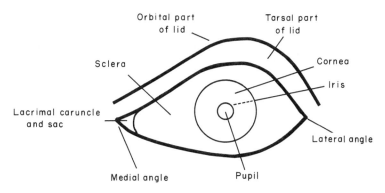

Fig. 8. The eye.

open, a distraught child and an overheated examiner. If
the child starts to cry when the light approaches his eye,
put the light away or let the child play with it and come
back to this part of the examination later. The sclera is
the white of the eye, the cornea the pigmented area. The
pupil is a designated area of the cornea. The clear area
of the cornea is round. A small pigmented curtain, the
iris, is normally also round and by constricting and re-
laxing, controls the amount of light which penetrates to
the retina. The space inside the iris is designated the
pupil (Fig. 8).

Vision may be tested roughly in the very young child
by noting the child's interest in a light or bright object and
noting the pupillary response to light. A newborn sees only
light, by one month can see smaller objects and by two
months can see rough outlines and follow moving fingers.
By six months, he should focus for short periods but is
farsighted. In an older child, vision can be estimated by
the child's interest in brightly colored objects in the room,
and the eye may be examined by having the child fix, if
even for a moment, on some familiar object such as the
parent's nose or face. Apparent blindness in a child less
than four months of age may be due to mental deficiency.

If more detailed tests of vision are desired, they
should be done before proceeding further with the examination of the eye. The infant can respond to light and

darkness and older children will cooperate when tested
with an eye chart. The infant may also be tested by rotating a cylinder on which black and white lines are painted.
An infant who sees will develop nystagmus as the cylinder
is rotated; the blind infant's eyes will remain stationary.
This is also a useful test in distinguishing hysterical from
organic blindness. The child of one to two years of age
may be noted as he picks up different-sized colored objects from the floor; the child of over two years of age
can usually be tested with a letter E chart, by asking the
child which way the bars point. Blindness or varying degrees of decreased visual acuity may be due to optic nerve
lesions, lesions anywhere in the eye including refractive
errors, or to cortical atrophy or central nervous system
defects. Occasionally, temporary blindness follows
head trauma with no sequelae. Unilateral visual defect
should focus one's attention to lesions peripheral to the
optic chiasm and in the eye.

   If there is any question of a brain lesion, visual
fields should be partially mapped. This is easily done in
a child over four years of age by confrontation. The examiner holds a piece of cotton in his hand, sits opposite
the child and has the child cover one eye while the examiner closes his eye. The child then looks at the examiner's open eye. The cotton is held at arm's length
and slowly brought in, in various planes midway between
the child and examiner toward their eyes. As soon as
the child sees the cotton, he will make a sudden move
toward it. This should occur at about the same time the
examiner sees the cotton. Younger children may be asked
to pick up small bright objects.

   Vertical defects are termed hemianopsias. Heter-
onymous defects are almost always bitemporal, due to
pressure on optic fibers at the chiasm. Homonymous
defects usually indicate lesions posterior to the chiasm
or in the visual cortex; temporal defects, lesions near
the chiasm. Sudden onset of blind spots, scotoma, which
enlarge and then resolve may be an early sign of migraine.
Central scotomas may be due to pressure on the chiasm
or to poisons. Constricted visual fields which are fixed

in size regardless of the distance from the patient may be caused by hysteria.

The next part of the routine eye examination consists in <u>observation</u> of the eye.

<u>Blinking</u> may be noted. Blinking normally occurs bilaterally when a quick movement is made toward the eyes or when one cornea is touched. This is the basis of the corneal reflex. Spasmodic blinking is usually due to habit spasm.

The <u>sclerae</u> should be completely white, but are blue in many normal children because of the normal thinness of the sclera. Blue sclerae are found in children with osteogenesis imperfecta and the Ehlers-Danlos syndrome. Yellow or mud-colored sclerae may be the first sign of clinical jaundice. In carotenemia, the skin is yellow but the sclerae are clear.

<u>Exophthalmos</u> and <u>enophthalmos</u> are noted. Exophthalmos is suspected if the eye appears large or protruding. Exophthalmos due to lid retraction occurs with hyperthyroidism, which is rare in childhood. It may be unilateral. The eyes may appear to bulge with congenital glaucoma or, rarely, glaucoma secondary to retrolental fibroplasia. The eyes may be pushed out, proptosis. Retro-orbital or orbital tumors or metastases, xanthomas of Hand-Schüller-Christian syndrome, neurofibromatosis, lymphangiomas, hemangiomas, and optic glioma may cause bulging. Orbital abscesses and sinus and cerebral thromboses, which are found especially in debilitated children with bacterial or fungal infections, may also cause bulging.

Enophthalmos is suspected if the eye appears sunken or small. Enophthalmos is usually due to cervical sympathetic nerve damage or microphthalmus, but apparent retraction of the eyeballs is observed in children with chronic malnutrition or acute dehydration.

The position of the eyes at rest should be noted. When the child looks straight ahead, the irises should be between the lids. The iris may appear to be beneath the lower lid, the "setting-sun" sign. This sign may be noted in normal prematures and sometimes in normal full-term infants. If marked, it is suggestive of hydrocephalus, increased intracranial pressure, or kernicterus.

Strabismus is noted. The eyes should be parallel when the child glances in any direction. If there is less parallelism when the eyes move in one direction, muscle paralysis is suspected. If the deviation from parallelism is equal when the eyes move in all directions the squint is non-paralytic or comitant. An easy method for observing squint is to look at the patient's eyes when he is looking toward a light about three feet away. The reflection of the light should come from approximately the same part of each pupil.

Degree of strabismus can be estimated by degree of deviation of the light reflection from the center of the pupils. Deviation is approximately 15 degrees if the reflection appears at the edge of the pupil, 30 degrees if the reflection is half-way between the edge of the pupil and the limbus (outer edge of the cornea), and 45 degrees if the reflection is at the edge of the limbus.

Another simple test for squint is the cover test. The examiner holds a light about two or three feet from the eyes, and sits directly in front of the patient. The patient is asked to focus on the light. One eye is then covered; the opposite eye is noted for motion. This eye is then covered and the first eye is noted for motion. Motion indicates the presence of strabismus or tropia. Eye dominance can be determined by noting which eye moves a little during the cover test. Resistance to covering one eye more than the other may be an indication of defective central vision in one eye.

Strabismus may be limited to one eye (monocular) or alternating. This can be determined by the constancy of the deviation in the cover test. Strabismus may be present only when the patient is tired, an intermittent squint. Test should also be made for strabismus with distant and near objects. Squint may be present for only one of these planes of focus, and still be comitant.

In children with paralytic strabismus, the involved eye does not complete the full range of motion. In non-paralytic strabismus each eye can move to all quadrants, but the eyes do not move simultaneously.

Paralytic strabismus is usually due to a lesion of the third, fourth, or sixth cranial nerves. Non-paralytic strabismus is usually due to muscle weakness, focusing difficulties, unilateral refractive error, non-fusion, or anatomical differences in the eyes. Vision should always be carefully checked in the presence of strabismus, especially for equality of vision in both eyes.

Strabismus is frequently present in the newborn, but should be minimal after six months of age. Even in the very young, however, fixed strabismus calls for a careful ophthalmological examination to exclude lesions which cause limitation of vision, such as optic atrophy, tumor, and chorioretinitis. Large epicanthic folds partly cover the globe of the eye and may be confused with squint. Paralytic, usually bilateral, internal strabismus may be an early sign of meningitis, increased intracranial pressure, and especially tuberculous meningitis. Paralytic strabismus also occurs with retrobulbar pain and otitis in children with petrositis.

Loss of upward gaze may be a sign of generalized increased intracranial pressure or of pineal tumor, or lesions in the superior colliculi (Parinaud's sign). Slow movements of the eyes may be observed with any condition causing paresis or paralysis of the eye muscles, or with hyperthyroidism.

Nystagmus is noted, usually by observing the constant motion of the eyes. Rarely, one attempts to induce horizontal nystagmus by having the patient focus on an object from the outer angle of the eye. The direction of the fast and slow components of the nystagmus should be recorded, as well as whether the nystagmus is spontaneous or induced.

In infancy, spontaneous nystagmus may occur in hypothyroidism or may be congenital, of unknown etiology. The infant may be blind and have a peculiar searching type of nystagmus. Nystagmus is characteristic of cerebellar lesions and brain tumors, and is also seen in the degenerative neurological diseases and vestibular diseases. It may be seen in children with severe refractive errors. Bilateral, asymmetrical nystagmus, pronounced in one eye and hardly discernible in the other, may be a sign of spasmus nutans. Nystagmus present with the eyes shut is congenital or should be considered vestibular in origin. Seesaw nystagmus, in which one eye moves rhythmically up while the other goes down, suggests a lesion near the third ventricle.

Ptosis of the lid may be congenital. It may represent birth injury to the brain or peripheral oculomotor nerve and, if associated with a sunken eyeball, constricted pupil, anhidrosis, and facial pallor, is due to cervical sympathetic paralysis (Horner's syndrome). Ptosis may be an early sign of myasthenia gravis and amyotonia congenita, and occurs in children with encephalitis or tendon injury to the levator palpebra superior. It may occasionally be noted in children recovering from tetany.

Only slight ptosis results from sympathetic paralysis. Third nerve paralysis results in severe ptosis. Ptosis associated with automatic elevation of the lid during chewing, the jaw-winking or Marcus Gunn phenomenon, is a congenital anomaly.

The palpebral fissures are more widely spaced on the involved side in children with facial palsy, because of weakness of the orbicularis oculi.

Other abnormalities of the eyelids should be noted. Hemorrhagic discoloration of the lids may be due to injury or to any of the bleeding dyscrasias such as scurvy or leukemia. Distortion of the lid may be due to edema, retrobulbar tumor, or metastases such as neuroblastoma. Extensive infection of the lids may be due to deep abscess formation or osteomyelitis around the sinuses. Fistulas near the lids may be congenital or may be due to chronic infection. Hemangiomas of the lids are very common. A violaceous hue may be noted in dermatomyositis and scleroderma.

Dark circles under the eyes may be noted. Their significance is uncertain, but may indicate tiredness, insufficient sleep, or allergy, or may be a residual of edema in the face.

The conjunctivae are examined for inflammation, conjunctivitis, hemorrhages and foreign body. Photophobia may be present with conjunctivitis. The usual

causes of redness of the conjunctivae in childhood are
bacterial or viral infection, allergy, measles or foreign
body. Conjunctivitis or hyperemia alone is also observed
in crying children and in children with eyestrain, emotional upsets, acrodynia, vitamin D poisoning, erythema
multiforme, and tridione sensitivity. An early sign of
measles, seen occasionally even before Koplik's spots in
the mouth, is the appearance of small red transverse lines
in the conjunctivae, Stimson's lines. Conjunctivitis in the
newborn is common and may be due to gonorrhea, chemical irritation or inclusion blenorrhea. It is well to note
the extent of the conjunctivitis. In gonorrheal conjunctivitis, the bulbar and palpebral conjunctivae are inflamed;
in conjunctivitis due to chemical irritation, usually the
bulbar conjunctiva is spared and only the palpebral conjunctiva is inflamed. A dry wrinkled conjunctiva with
foamy yellow patches, Bitot's spots, occurs in children
with vitamin A deficiency. Small comma-shaped vessels
in the lower bulbar conjunctivae are characteristic of
vascular stasis and sickle-cell disease.

Small hemorrhages in the conjunctivae may be
cardinal signs of bacterial endocarditis, scurvy or meningococcemia. They are also seen in the bleeding diseases. They are commonly seen in the normal newborn
and are common in children following cough or trauma.

Pingueculae are small, yellowish wedge-shaped
areas near the cornea. They occasionally occur with the
xanthomatoses or Gaucher's disease. Pterygium, a
wing-shaped white area which may cover the cornea, is
an extension of the conjunctiva.

Styes (hordeolum) are seen usually on the lower lid
as tender, reddish-yellow pustules at the root of the hair
follicle. Recurrent styes may be a sign of eyestrain,
exposure to dust or dirt, general debility, or hay fever,
though a stye may be an early sign of diabetes. A non-
painful yellow swelling of the lid edge is due to inclusion
cyst, chalazion. Scaling of the lid margins, blepharitis,
may be due to seborrhea, allergy, or infection.

The cornea is best examined with good room illumination or with an open bulb about two feet in front of the

patient. It should be crystal clear. Any inflammation, ulceration, or opacity is abnormal.

Redness of the cornea due to vessel engorgement is noted. If the redness is less near the cornea and increases toward the conjunctiva, superficial inflammation, keratitis, is probably present; if redness is greater near the cornea and fades toward the periphery, deep (ciliary) inflammation is present.

Opacities in the cornea usually are due to ulcerations. Yellow opacities usually indicate active ulcerations, while bluish-white opacities are healed ulcerations. Depth of ulceration should be noted. Active ulcerations are usually associated with pain, photophobia, redness of the eye and a small pupil. If inflammation or opacity is present, foreign body, trauma or infection should be suspected. Corneal ulceration may occur with riboflavin deficiency or may be due to herpes.

Pinhead grayish ulcerations with conjunctivitis or phlyctenular keratoconjunctivitis is a rare painful form of tuberculosis or tuberculin sensitivity. It begins at the corneal-scleral junction, then invades the cornea. Deep ciliary inflammation is especially common in children with interstitial keratitis due to late congenital syphilis. The whole cornea may appear steamy white. Keratoconjunctivitis also occurs with measles and other viral diseases, and with rheumatoid arthritis. A gray-green-orange ring around the cornea, the Kayser-Fleischer ring, is seen in hepatolenticular degeneration, Wilson's disease.

Haziness of the cornea is found in children with glaucoma, avitaminosis A, and diseases with hypercholesteremia. It may also be seen in children with such metabolic diseases as gargoylism and cystinosis, though usually slit-lamp examination is necessary to demonstrate crystal formation in the cornea. A large cornea may also be a sign of glaucoma.

Foreign bodies on the cornea or conjunctiva may be detected easily unless they lie over the pupil. If foreign body is suspected, the lids should be everted and the light should be swung in different directions, as careful examination is made. Either the foreign body or its shadow

will be observed. The lids can be everted by asking the
patient to look down, placing an applicator stick just over
the edge of the upper eyelid and pulling the eyelid forward
and upward. If a suspected foreign body cannot be located,
fluorescein sticks may be placed in the eye. On oblique
illumination, the injured area of the cornea will stand out
with a greenish fluorescence.

With the light in the same position the anterior chamber may be noted. Blood or small white spots may be observed. Blood is usually due to injury. White spots may
be an early sign of uveitis.

Discharges from the eye should be noted. An infant
ordinarily does not have tears before one month of age,
and the lacrimal duct opens several weeks later. A watery
discharge in infancy, usually from one eye, may signify a
blocked tear duct. Pressure should be made on the tear
sac, just below the inner canthus of the eye. At the same
time, the lower lid should be slightly everted so that the
small opening (punctum) can be observed. If fluid escapes
when pressure is applied, obstruction below the lacrimal
sac may exist. Fixed red painful swelling and induration
in the area of the lacrimal sac indicate abscess formation
with blockage, dacryocystitis. Obstruction without infection is usually a congenital anomaly; with infection, an
acquired disease. Tearing with a wet nose, however,
may be a sign of infantile glaucoma; with a blocked tear
duct, the nose is usually dry.

Watery discharges, epiphora, are seen also with
allergy, sinusitis, and styes. Purulent discharges are
due to infections; in the newborn period the pus due to
the chemical irritants placed in the eye may easily be
confused with gonorrheal ophthalmia. Absence of tears
has been noted as a characteristic of children with familial
autonomic dysfunction.

The pupils are compared for size and shape. They
should be round, regular, clear, and equal. Irregulari-
ties in the pupil are usually due to congenital malformations. The sudden appearance of an irregular pupil should
make one immediately suspect a penetrating foreign body
through the cornea. White bands over the pupil may be
due to congenitally persistent pupillary membranes. Un-

equal pupils, anisocoria, are usually congenital, but if they appear suddenly in the presence of equal illumination, usually indicate acute intracranial disease.

Reaction to light of the pupils is noted. Size and light reaction are controlled by the sympathetic nervous system and the parasympathetics carried by the 3rd cranial nerve. Children's pupils should react to light quickly. Reaction of the pupil in which the light shines is the direct reaction; of the opposite pupil, consensual reaction. The pupils of newborn infants are constricted until about the third week of age so that light reaction, while always sluggish in an infant with congenital glaucoma, is not a good test of glaucoma in the newborn. Sympathetic nervous stimulation causes dilatation; parasympathetic, constriction. Acute pain may cause dilatation of pupils.

A fixed dilated pupil indicates sympathetic stimulation, blindness, or poisoning. It may be caused by pressure on the midbrain due to acute increase in intracranial pressure. It may indicate a homolateral extradural or subdural hematoma, or meningitis. Dilated unreactive pupils are seen also with atropine or deep barbiturate poisoning or anoxia. Coma and acidosis cause dilated pupils. The pupils do not react in children whose coma is due to compressing lesions of the brain; they usually are reactive in comatose children with metabolic disease. The pupils remain dilated in children with partial blindness, but the pupils respond to light in children with cortical blindness.

Constricted unreactive pupils are seen in children with cervical sympathetic palsy (Horner's syndrome), or in children with opiate, light barbiturate, or cholinesterase enzyme poisoning. In neurosyphilis of childhood the pupils remain fixed and small due to parasympathetic injury. Constricted pupils generally indicate that the third nerve impulses are intact.

Hippus is exaggerated rhythmic contraction and dilation of the pupils. It may be a normal variant, but also occurs with central nervous system disease.

Accommodation can be tested even in small children by having them look first at a shiny colored object at a distance and quickly bringing the object toward the eye.

The pupil contracts as the object is brought near the eye
and this reaction is known as the convergence reaction.
Various neurological disorders, including diphtheria,
cause loss of the accommodation reflex. Most infants are
hyperopic, but occasionally a very young infant will play
with objects within two or three inches of his face. He will
probably be myopic when vision becomes fully developed.

The iris is usually blue at birth and becomes pigmented within six months. Inequality of pigmentation may
be a congenital anomaly or may be due to metallic foreign
bodies. In Horner's syndrome the involved side remains
blue while the opposite side acquires pigment. Different
colored irises may indicate Waardenburg's syndrome.
The iris is observed to determine any fluttering, which
may occur with subluxation or detachment of the lens.
Absence of a part of the iris may be noted, as in colo-
boma; it may be associated with Wilms' tumor. Adhesions may be seen from the iris toward the lens. These
may be congenital, due to persistence of the pupillary
membranes, or may occur with chronic iritis, as in
rheumatoid arthritis. Black and white spots in the iris
are usually seen in children with mongolism. Nodules
may be seen in the iris due to tuberculosis. When a
light shines on the iris, the eye lights up as if a switch
was thrown, in albinism.

The lens is examined with direct light from the un-
shaded bulb. White or gray spots usually indicate opacities, cataracts in the lens. The usual causes of cataracts in newborn infants are rubella in the mother during
the first trimester of pregnancy, congenital cataracts of
unknown cause, hypoparathyroidism, glaucoma in the infant, or galactosemia. With cataract, almost nothing can
be seen beyond the white membrane of the lens when the
light shines into the eye (Fig. 9).

Successful internal examination of the eye depends
on having gained the confidence of the child, and having
learned to develop a picture image of what one sees in a
flash. This same technique is useful in the examination
of the pharynx of the child. The room should be darkened
and the patient should be told that the room will be darken-

TEMPORAL

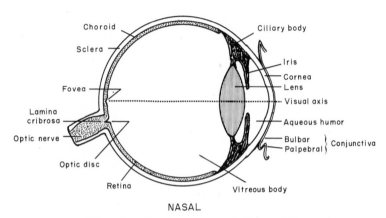

NASAL

Fig. 9. Section through the orbit.

ed, that a light will shine in his eyes, but that nothing painful will be done. Eye drops should be avoided but may be necessary. If the child is old enough, he is asked to look at a brightly colored picture across the room. The somewhat younger child can be given your flashlight and asked to turn it on and shine it on the picture across the room.

First, one uses a +8 -- +2 lens to examine the cornea, iris and lens and then an 0 -- -2 lens is used for examination of the disc and retina. The examiner should use his right eye to examine the patient's right eye, and his left eye for the patient's left eye. The examiner starts about a foot away from the patient's eye, and as he approaches the eye, he changes the ophthalmoscope lenses so that they become less positive. The retina (Fig. 10) is usually best visible with an 0 -- -2 lens in infants and children, and is usually seen first as a red area, the red reflex, and then the details become obvious. Opacities in the cornea, anterior chamber or lens will usually be seen with this type of illumination as black spots against the red reflex of the retina. Their significance has already

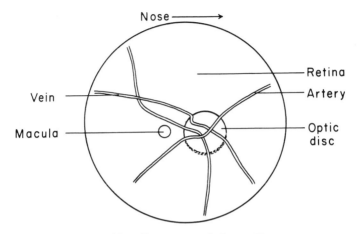

Fig. 10. Diagram of the retina.

been described. With direct light, pearly gray, opaque, round areas in the center of the lens are typical of cataracts. Lenticular cataracts are usually lamellar (zonular) in children. The lens may appear clear but out of shape. The posterior eye structures will be seen with difficulty. The lens may be seen dislocated upward, as in Marfan's syndrome, or downward, as in patients with homocystinuria.

The appearance of the red reflex alone from the retina is important information. Ordinarily, the fundus will be pink and shiny, but may be gray in deeply pigmented or in anemic children. The retina becomes gray and loses its shine whenever it becomes avascular. Absence of the red reflex or the appearance of a white-opaque membrane is noted in those children with opacities of the cornea, lens, cataracts, persistent posterior fibrovascular sheath of the lens, retrolental fibroplasia, retinal detachment or retinoblastoma.

Veins and arteries are noted to be of almost equal caliber, or the veins are slightly larger than the arteries. Narrow arteries are seen in the hypertensive diseases, especially nephritis. The vessels are dilated and cyanotic in children with cyanotic heart disease. Venous distention is an early sign of increased intracranial pressure. The veins are noted to pulsate normally. Exaggerated pulsations of the arteries, however, may indicate arteriovenous fistula, aortic regurgitation or other causes of increased pulse pressure. All of the vessels of the disc are engorged with inflammation of the optic nerve, optic neuritis, and may appear small and thickened with arteritis, as in the collagen diseases.

Fresh hemorrhages on the retina in the newborn may indicate only trauma or anoxia or may be a cardinal sign of subdural hematoma. They appear as red spots or as red spots with a surrounding white haze. These spots are also seen with sinus thrombosis, leukemia, scurvy, bacterial endocarditis and other bleeding diseases. Multiple gray mulberry-like tubercles in the retina are seen in children with tuberous sclerosis, tuberculosis, or neurofibromatosis.

Patchy areas of white and red indicate chorioretinitis. They may appear in various infections but are characteristic of infection with toxoplasmosis, cytomegalic inclusion disease, syphilis, tuberculosis, and chronic brucellosis. Grayish-brown streaks radiating out from the disc are angioid, seen in pseudoxanthoma elasticum.

The disc is most easily found if the examiner relaxes and gazes from the temporal side of the patient's eye toward the posterior aspects of the eye. The edges of the disc usually have a sharp border around half the circumference and then fade. Blurring should be noted. The entire disc may be surrounded by a melanin ring. This is usually normal. Gray stippling around the optic disc is a sign of lead poisoning. The disc is usually in the same plane as the retina in childhood. It is usually a little less pink than the surrounding retina. It is very pale in patients with anemia.

Bruit over the eyeball may occur with congenital arteriovenous fistulas in the brain.

The disc may appear large and swollen, the edges may appear blurred, and the retinal vessels may appear

to bend down from the disc to the retina in children with
papilledema. Such "choked" or bulging discs indicate increased intracranial pressure or optic neuritis. Brain
tumors or abscesses, except those originating in the anterior fossa, usually cause papilledema. Pulmonary insufficiency may be associated with papilledema. The disc
appears white in children with optic neuritis or optic
atrophy, and may be seen in children with meningitis,
encephalitis, many other generalized infections, cystic
fibrosis, especially those receiving chloramphenicol,
many types of poisonings, thiamine deficiency, brain
tumors, optic nerve tumors, fibrous dysplasia, congenital syphilis, or neurofibroma. It may precede other
signs of multiple sclerosis, or it may be an isolated
finding. Unilateral papilledema with contralateral optic
atrophy may be due to a frontal lobe tumor, Foster
Kennedy syndrome. If the retina appears opalescent,
retinal detachment may be present.

Cupping of the disc in which the vessels appear to
dip down from the retina toward the disc may be physiological or may be exaggerated with glaucoma. A white
disc may indicate optic nerve atrophy, as occurs with
osteopetrosis causing compression of the nerve, or with
neurofibroma of the optic nerve. It also occurs following
optic neuritis which affects the nerve far back of the eyeball, as with multiple sclerosis or methyl alcohol poisoning.

Just to the temporal side of the disc is a small yellow-
red area devoid of vessels, the macula. Since this is the
most light-sensitive area of the eye, the pupil constricts
as the macula is approached. In older children, the macula can be visualized if the patient is told to look at the
ophthalmoscope light. This area appears to be cherry-red
in reticuloendothelial diseases such as Tay-Sachs and
Niemann-Pick disease or in other cerebromacular degenerative diseases. The macula may be brown and
appear fragmented in children with the juvenile form of
macular degeneration.

Late in the examination the corneal reflex should be
obtained by touching the cornea with a piece of cotton. Both
eyes normally shut. Failure to obtain the corneal reflex

indicates trigeminal (sensory component) or facial (motor component) nerve injury. Pontine injuries and anesthesia depress this reflex.

In general, complete cooperation is impossible with young children. As the child gets older, devices for obtaining attention should be used. However, with or without cooperation, the areas of the eye listed should be explored. If a defect is noted in any of these areas, the patient should be referred to an ophthalmologist, who can use other instruments and anesthetics.

EARS

Except for the thermolabile children, the commonest cause of fever without obvious reason in childhood is ear infection. Obviously, the ears of all sick children should be examined.

Various anomalies of the ears occur (Fig. 11). These are usually obvious deformities of the auricle and

Fig. 11. The external ear.

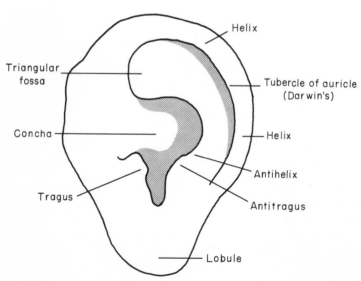

are not listed. Occasionally, a small sinus is present
as a hole or pit just in front of the ear, and may be accompanied by a small swelling just inside the canal; this
represents the remnant of the first branchial cleft.

The position of the ears is noted. In a rare anomaly
in the newborn, the tops of the ears are below the level of
the eye and there is congenital absence of the kidneys
(Potter's syndrome). Other gross anomalies of the ears
may be associated with lesser kidney anomalies.

The auricles frequently appear to stand forward with
any mass or swelling behind the ear. Important conditions
causing this appearance are mastoiditis, cellulitis, mumps
and postauricular abscesses. Occasionally, enlarged post-
auricular nodes or external otitis with surrounding cellulitis makes the ears protrude.

The nature and odor of discharge from the aural
canals is noted. A greenish foul-smelling discharge occurs with pyocyaneus infections. Purulent discharges
are seen with any bacterial infection, particularly pneu-
mococcus and M. tuberculosis, but may also occur with
fungal infections of the canal wall. Generalized eczema
may cause flaking in the ears. Bloody discharge is
usually due to scratching, irritation or injury of the ear
canal but may occur with foreign body in the canal or be
a cardinal sign of basilar skull fracture.

Next, the otoscope is used (Fig. 12). Several points
should be remembered about the otoscope. First, it should
be operating properly and the batteries should be fresh,
lest the light be yellow. Second, the largest possible
speculum should be used. The speculum must be cleaned
before use and need never enter the canal more than one-
quarter inch, or one-half inch in the older child. The only
use for the one- or two-millimeter speculum, even in infants, is to cloud the field and hurt the patient. Third,
the canal should be examined before one tries to look at
the drum. This is not for fear of missing something as
much as it is to note the presence of a furuncle or vesicle
in the outer edge of the canal. Jam the otoscope on a
furuncle once and the examination is ended! Fourth, the
otoscope should be held firmly with one hand and, as the
speculum is inserted, the hand holding the otoscope should

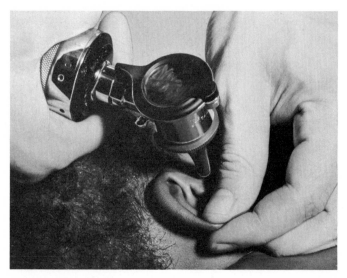

Fig. 12. Using the otoscope. The hand holding the otoscope rests firmly on the patient's head or face.

rest firmly on the patient's head or face so that any motion by the patient will be accompanied by a similar movement of the otoscope. Fifth, it is frequently valuable to place the speculum just inside the canal of one ear then the other before attempting to examine the drum. This assures the patient that the procedure will not hurt. Finally, before using the otoscope the direction of the canal must be remembered. In the infant, the canal is directed upward, so the auricle should be pulled down to view the drum. In the older child, the canal faces downward and forward, so the tip of the auricle is pulled up and back for adequate visualization. Pulling the external ear serves another useful purpose. Ordinarily, this movement is painless, and it is painless in children with otitis media; but it is painful in children with a furuncle in the ear or external otitis.

Examination of the ears should be almost painless. The child should be allowed to play with the otoscope, but at the time of the examination he should be handled firmly.

Either the child assures the examiner of cooperation, or the mother holds him so that the head does not move and the hands do not interfere. The child should be placed face down, prone, with the head turned first to one side, then the other. Tell him that he is going to hear a song through the speculum. He must be very quiet. After the first ear, ask if he heard the song. Then do the same in the opposite ear.

The canal is examined. The canal and auricle may be swollen in children with external otitis, as occurs with seborrhea, allergic dermatitis, or in nervous children who frequently place foreign bodies in the canal. Any tenderness is noted. Tenderness as the speculum is placed in the canal may indicate disease of the canal, such as a furuncle, or disease of the middle ear, otitis media. Vesicles in the canal may be due to viral canal infections or otitis media caused by H. influenzae. If cerumen is present, frequently a large enough speculum allows one to look above or below the wax at the drum. If a small, easily reached foreign body or obstructive wax is present, it is best removed with an ear spoon or wire loop.

Discharges may arise from the canal, external otitis, from otitis media with perforation of the drum, or from chronic otitis media with mastoiditis. Swimmer's discharge is usually due to gram-negative bacilli. Greenish discharge is usually from external otitis. Mucoid or mucopurulent discharge most often arises from the middle ear.

Discharges should be carefully wiped away with a soft cotton-tipped applicator. Care must be used to blot the discharge so as not to push anything against an ear drum which may be perforated. Cotton-tipped applicators should not be used for removing hard wax or foreign bodies.

One may rarely resort to the use of an ear syringe to remove adherent wax. The wax should first be softened with a detergent. The syringe should be fitted with a narrow "fistula tip" to provide a thin stream. It is then filled with lukewarm water (the patient is covered to prevent soaking), and is introduced gently into the tip of the canal, which is then flushed. This procedure is unpleasant and undesirable in examining children because a vestibular response, frequently with vomiting, is induced. It should

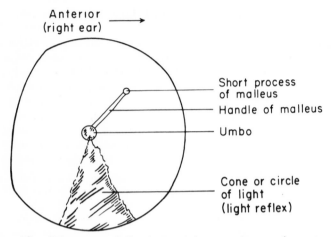

Fig. 13.   Diagram of the tympanic membrane (ear drum).

never be done if a perforation of the drum is suspected, or if a foreign body is in the canal.

The normal drum (Fig. 13) is gray-white and trans-lucent or opalescent.   The handle of the malleus appears as a small white streak running down and back to the center of the ear and ends at the umbo.   At the upper end of the malleus is a small white projection, the short process of the malleus.   Below the umbo is a small circle of light, the light reflex.   Even in the infant, whose drum is almost horizontal, these landmarks should be determined.   As the child gets older, the drum becomes vertical but points in-ward.   The light reflex becomes cone-shaped and sharply outlined with the apex at the center and the base at the an-terior inferior portion of the drum.

The most common abnormality of the drum that is noted on otoscopic examination is slight redness.   This may be due to crying or to manipulation.   If the drum is slightly to markedly reddened, the vessels prominent, and retracted as noted by the prominence of the malleus and a deeper and sharper outline of the cone of light, catarrhal otitis media is present.   This is usually due to any upper respiratory infection or to obstruction of the eustachian tube. The light reflex may appear less prominent than usual.

In acute suppurative otitis media, the <u>light reflex</u> is usually lost; the drum bulges outward and becomes diffusely red; the handle of the malleus is not seen clearly, and hearing is usually decreased. Occasionally, with a bulging drum, the light reflex instead of being lost is scattered diffusely over the drum area. The examiner must recognize that this reflex is coming from a convex drum, as the handle of the malleus is not seen. Otitis media in the young infant may be due to congenital syphilis in addition to the usual causes of suppuration, such as <u>H. influenzae</u>, pneumococci, streptococci, staphylococci and viruses. Otitis, sometimes with mastoiditis, and abducens paralysis of the homolateral eye occur with petrositis, Gradenigo's syndrome. Chronic otitis may be due to tuberculosis as well as to other bacteria and may be associated with enlarged adenoids or mastoiditis. Otitis in the infant may be caused by the infant having been fed frequently by propping the bottle or in the supine position.

Bulging also may be due to non-purulent fluid. This may be noted in children with late catarrhal otitis media or with suppurative otitis in whom the bacterial infection has resolved but before the exudate has been resorbed, serous otitis. Bulging with a bluish discoloration of the drum may be due to a collection of blood in the middle ear and occurs after trauma and sometimes after infection. Blood behind the drum suggests basilar skull fracture.

The drum may be <u>perforated</u>. Perforation with pus indicates acute or chronic purulent otitis media. Small perforations may be seen in the drum due to injury, insect bites or chronic tuberculosis.

Varying degrees of redness of the drum with possibly some loss of the light reflex, but without bulging or retraction and without evidence of fluid in the middle ear, especially if accompanied by exquisite pain and little hearing loss, may indicate myringitis. Myringitis is a primary inflammation of the drum head without involvement of the middle ear, or it may be an early stage of otitis media.

Occasionally, one sees a small mass, usually gray, red or yellow, just in front of or behind the drum, from which pus oozes. This is termed a cholesteatoma. A pinpoint perforation may accompany it in the posterior superior or central portion of the drum.

Mobility of the drum is noted. This requires a tight fitting otoscope and speculum with a small hole through which a puff of air can be introduced with an attached rubber bulb. The light reflex and drum will be seen to move. An immovable drum is found in suppurative or serous otitis media. Serous otitis is a condition with conductive hearing loss with a fluid-like secretion in the middle ear. It may be caused by allergies, chronic infections, hypothyroidism, obesity, or anything that contributes to the closure of the eustachian tube. An immovable drum also is found in children with osteopetrosis.

Next, one feels and taps the mastoid tip of the temporal bone. Any fluctuation or tenderness is noted; either may indicate mastoiditis.

Just behind the mastoid, one feels for the postauricular nodes. In a child these are normally about 1 or 2 mm. in diameter. Enlarged nodes are characteristic of German measles, nits or inflammation of the scalp, and are usually slightly tender. They are also found in children with measles, roseola, varicella, infectious mononucleosis, leukemia or tick bites. In this area, also, one occasionally feels subcutaneous nodules, about 2-5 mm. in diameter. These nodules are characteristic of active rheumatic fever.

Hearing is estimated. In a small child, this can best be tested by making a sharp noise at the child's ear and noting a blinking of the eyes. Each ear is tested separately with the examiner standing outside the direct line of vision of the child. In an older child, it is sufficient to test the whispered voice at about eight feet. This is best done by asking the child simple questions or whispering a simple command. Nothing is quite so gratifying as diagnosing impaired hearing in a child who was thought to be mentally defective. Many children will tell you they hear a watch tick when it is held about 6 to 10 inches from the

head. The doctor can develop this into a relatively quan-
titative hearing test after using his watch with a small
number of normal children and determining how far from
the ear the watch can be heard.

Loss of hearing can be conductive, neurosensory
or mixed. Over the age of three most mentally normal
children are cooperative enough to be tested with a tuning
fork. The tip of the vibrating tuning fork is pressed
against the mastoid process of the child, then of the
examiner. The number of seconds it is heard by both
is compared. If the child hears it for less time than the
examiner, this indicates decreased bone conduction, a
sign of neurosensory hearing loss. If he hears it longer,
this indicates conductive loss (Schwabach test). Air and
bone conduction can be compared in the patient. First
the fork is placed on the mastoid as before, then about
one inch from the ear with approximately equal vibratory
stimulus. Normally, air conduction is twice as long as
bone conduction (Rinne). The vibrating fork is then
placed on the middle of the child's forehead, and he is
asked in which ear he hears it better. In unilateral conductive deafness, the hearing is better in the unaffected
side (Weber test). In unilateral neurosensory deafness,
the hearing is better in the affected ear.

Hearing loss may be due simply to foreign body or
cerumen in the canals. Defective hearing may be noted in
children with chronic catarrhal otitis media associated
with enlarged adenoids or other nasal obstruction, in children who have received dihydrostreptomycin, or in children who have had meningitis, encephalitis, kernicterus,
or gargoylism. Congenital deafness is usually idiopathic,
or it may be found in children whose mothers had rubella
during the first trimester of pregnancy. Unilateral deafness may follow mumps. Deafness associated with syncope
may be due to congenital heart lesions, Jervell and Lange-
Nielsen syndrome. Deafness may be associated with hereditary renal disease with hyperprolinemia or with a
white forelock and eye abnormalities in Waardenburg's
syndrome. Pseudodeafness may be seen in psychotic
children, especially those with autism, or in children

with mental deficiency. More complicated types of deafness should be referred to an otologist. Hyperacute
hearing may be seen in children with Tay-Sachs disease
or tetanus.

Children who have received streptomycin or who
have nystagmus or an unsteady gait should have their
vestibular function tested. The cold caloric test usually
suffices. The patient is seated and water of 65 F. is in-
jected into the ear. Nystagmus should appear within 30
seconds. Alternatively the child may be rotated. The
examiner rapidly rotates the child around himself 3 or 4
times. Nystagmus normally occurs. The absence of
nystagmus indicates vestibular or brain stem disease.
This may be due to streptomycin, labyrinthitis, meningitis
or brain tumor or a sign of benign paroxysmal vertigo.

NOSE

Examination of the nose, even superficially, is often
neglected. Yet not too rarely it holds the key to the proper
diagnosis.

Any unusual shape of the nose is noted. Because the
lower half of the nasal septum is cartilage, one rarely sees
fracture or dislocation of the nose in childhood. Deviation
occasionally is seen in the newborn, perhaps due to intrauterine position. The chief cause of flattening of the nose
in childhood is cleft palate. With cleft palate the nasal
septum is deflected and the nose appears flattened. A
saddle-shaped nose is characterized by a low bridge and
broad base. This is usually seen as a familial characteristic but also occurs in children with hypertelorism or
following perforation of the septum, as in congenital
syphilis.

Flaring of the alae nasi should be noted. The alae
flare with all types of respiratory obstruction or distress,
but particularly with pneumonia. Flaring of the alae nasi
may be seen in children with fevers, acidosis, peritonitis
or any condition or illness causing anoxia.

Next, one shines a light up the nose and the color of
the mucosa is noted. If the tip of the nose is pushed upward with the thumb of the left hand, and the light is held

with the right hand, one can frequently observe high into the nose. A speculum is usually not necessary for satisfactory examination of the mucosa or the ostia of the sinuses. If a nasal speculum is desired, one should use the spring-type rather than the otoscope speculum. The large otoscope speculum may be placed in the tip of the nose and the area up to the middle meatus may be examined. The nasal speculum is preferably used with a head mirror, but satisfactory examination can be performed with a hand light if the mother holds the baby's head firmly. A red, inflamed mucosa indicates infection. A pale, boggy mucosa may indicate allergy. A swollen grayish mucosa may indicate chronic rhinitis.

The character of secretions should be noted. Purulent secretions are common with any nasal infection, even the usual upper respiratory infection in its later stages, or may be an early sign of the contagious diseases, particularly measles, pertussis or poliomyelitis. Purulent secretions from the ostia above or below the middle turbinates indicate sinusitis; pus in the middle meatus suggests involvement of the maxillary, frontal, or anterior ethmoid sinuses; in the superior meatus, involvement of the posterior ethmoid or sphenoid sinuses. Patients with discharge and crusting below or on the edges of the alae nasi, particularly with redness of the surrounding skin, usually have infections with β-hemolytic streptococci. Purulent discharges may also be caused by H. influenzae or pneumococci. Purulent or bloody secretions in infancy may be a sign of secondary syphilis. When due to syphilis, they may occur up to the age of six months and are usually associated with excoriations of the upper lip.

Watery nasal secretions may indicate allergy, the common cold, foreign bodies high in the nose or, rarely, skull fracture or perforated encephalocele. Unilateral purulent secretions suggest foreign body, nasal diphtheria, nasal polyps or sinusitis.

Bleeding points in the nose should be noted. They are most commonly found at the lower anterior tip of the septum.

Epistaxis is rare in infancy and if present may in-

dicate a bleeding dyscrasia. The usual cause of epistaxis,
hemoptysis or hematemesis in children is irritation or injury of the nasal mucosa, and is especially common in
children with allergic rhinitis. Other less common causes
of epistaxis include nasal infections, particularly diphtheria;
typhoid fever, leukemia, rheumatic fever, foreign body,
and congestion due to any cause such as congenital heart
disease. Occasionally, epistaxis in childhood is caused
by late syphilis, elevated blood pressure due to any cause,
or any of the anemias or bleeding diseases. Bleeding after
skull injury may be due to local nasal injury or to skull
fracture. Rarely, a bleeding telangiectasis is seen in the
mucosa and may be the cardinal sign of familial telan-
giectasia. Epistaxis may be the only physical sign of hereditary hemorrhagic thrombasthenia, one of the bleeding
diseases.

Note should be made of the child's ability to get air
through the nose. Infection, foreign body, vasomotor
rhinitis, tumor, polyp or a badly deviated septum are the
usual causes of inability to breathe through the nose. The
newborn with bilateral choanal atresia is unable to get air
through his nostrils and often appears to be choking. In
the older child, large adenoids, even if uninfected, may
cause nasal obstruction with a typical adenoid facies.

An unusually large nasal airway with dry crusting
is occasionally noted. This may be a sign of atrophic
rhinitis, which occurs in older children or adults; a mal-
odorous nasal discharge may be present.

In the older child, the nasal septum should be examined. Perforation may be due to injury of the nasal
septum, foreign body, syphilis or tuberculosis. The
nasal septum is deflected in children with cleft palate.
Otherwise, septal deviations are rare in childhood.

Occasionally polyps or tumors may occlude one of
the nostrils or even protrude from the nose. Polyps frequently occur with allergy, but may be a manifestation of
chronic infection, cystic fibrosis, or generalized polyposis. An encephalocele may protrude through the cribri-
form plate and appear to be a polyp. A membrane in the
nose preceded by bleeding should be considered diphtheria
until this diagnosis can be eliminated.

The sinus areas should be percussed as previously described for evidence of pain. The maxillary and ethmoid sinuses are developed in infancy, and the frontal sinuses by five to seven years. Transillumination of the sinuses is generally unsatisfactory in childhood.

Olfactory nerve tests are generally not done in childhood.

THROAT

Examination of the mouth and throat is usually deferred to the end of the examination. In order to see adequately the posterior pharynx and particularly the epiglottis during gagging, it is essential that the child be sitting. He must either be cooperative or adequately restrained when the depressor is finally placed far back in the mouth. Preferably the patient is in the sitting position during this entire part of the examination. If the mother or an assistant is present, the child should be set on this person's lap. The mother or assistant is asked to hold both the child's wrists with one hand and the forehead with the other (see Fig. 15). The very young may be restrained and examined supine (Fig. 14).

As in the examination of the fundus of the eye, a photographic memory is helpful. In many children, a brief glimpse of the interior of the mouth is all that one may obtain. It is usually helpful to give a child a tongue depressor while the examination is proceeding. Then the examiner asks the child to open his mouth while the child holds the tongue depressor. First the external structures are examined.

Around the mouth, circumoral pallor is noted. With circumoral pallor the immediate area around the mouth appears white, while a strip just below the nose, the surface of the cheeks and the lower chin are red. This appearance may occur with any febrile disease, but it is particularly noted in children who have just exercised or who have scarlet or rheumatic fever or hypoglycemia. Even in infants with seborrheic dermatitis and eczema, though the remainder of the cheeks may be covered with scales this pale area usually remains free of lesions.

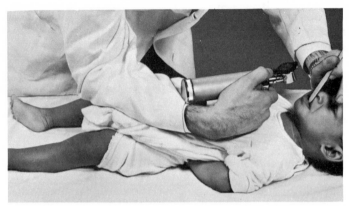

Fig. 14. Restraining the patient for examination of the mouth. Patient's arms are tucked under his back. Examiner's hand presses on chest and holds light. Examiner's other hand holds patient's head and tongue depressor.

The lips are inspected. Asymmetry of the mouth with twisting of the lips to one side is found with facial nerve or trigeminal nerve paralysis. Cleft lip, usually on the left side, is a congenital anomaly. Extent and location of the cleft should be noted. Lip pits may appear as isolated deformities or associated with other anomalies.

Slight fissures of the lips, cheilitis, are frequently seen in children exposed to wind and sun. Rhagades, however, are deep fissures or their resultant scars coming from the nose to the lips and extending outward from the lips. They are characteristic of congenital syphilis. Deep radiating painful fissures from the ends of the lips, cheilosis, are seen in numerous nutritional disturbances, particularly riboflavin and other B-vitamin deficiencies, or with Monilia or other infections. Excoriation of the upper lip occurs frequently in young children with simple upper respiratory infections.

Vesicles and pustules appear on the lips in older children, especially following upper respiratory infections. "Cold sores" or herpes simplex are vesicles on an inflamed base and usually burn or itch. Bacterial infections are detected as ordinary pustules. Retention cysts, usually single, occur on the lip and appear as small protrusions containing clear fluid.

The color of the lips is noted. The normal pink color of white children or gray of the Negro is replaced by a pale mucosa when anemia is present. Gray cyanosis is seen with most congenital heart lesions, methemoglobinemia, anoxia and bizarre poisons. Deep purple lips are seen with severe congenital heart disease. Cherry-red lips are characteristically seen in infants and children with acidosis, frequently due to aspirin poisoning or diabetes in the older child. Cherry-red lips are also seen in patients with carbon monoxide poisoning. With many poisons the lips may appear red while the remainder of the body is pallid.

The lips may be grossly swollen due to insect bites, local infection or injury, angioneurotic edema or massive generalized edema.

Unusual odors from the mouth should be noted. The sweetish odor of acetone is common in dehydrated or malnourished children, but may indicate diabetic acidosis as in adults. A mouse-like odor occurs in children with diphtheria. A peculiar odor similar to that obtained from decaying tissue may occur in children with typhoid fever. An ammoniacal odor occurs in children with uremia. Halitosis, or bad breath, occurs in children with many varied states including poor local hygiene, local or systemic infections, sinusitis and mouth-breathing.

It is useless to ask a child less than six or seven years of age if his throat hurts, for even with acute pharyngitis or tonsillitis, the child usually has no pain. Pain in the younger child, if present, more commonly indicates the presence of epiglottis or laryngitis, or occasionally abscess, diphtheria, or scarlatina.

Most patients will open their mouths when asked to do so. Inability of a child to open his mouth is generally only voluntary and not a real inability. Real inability to open the mouth occurs with tetanus (trismus), tetany, infections in the tissues surrounding the mouth, dislocation of the temporomandibular joint and, occasionally, parotitis. Rarely, in rheumatic fever or rheumatoid arthritis, the swollen temporomandibular joint prevents the patient from opening his mouth. Ankylosis of the joint may occur rarely secondary to birth injury to the joint. Temporomandibular joint involvement can frequently be recognized not only by the apparent inability to move the joint, but also by obvious asymmetry of the face. Trismus may also occur in children with infantile Gaucher's disease, brain tumor and encephalitis, and is noted frequently in children who receive phenothiazine derivatives.

If the child does not open his mouth after suggestion, he may be told to show his teeth. If he declines, the tongue blade is placed gently between the lips and the mucosa is pushed away from the teeth to obtain an adequate view of the teeth, gums and mucosa. If mouth lesions are suspected, it is frequently less painful if the tongue blade is moistened before insertion. Only if the patient moves is he restrained. Sometimes, in older children, if one pushes down first one side of the tongue, then the other, it is easier to visualize all the mouth and throat. Good lighting, preferably daylight, is necessary for further examination. It is important, however, to become accustomed to the use of one type of light, either daylight or electric. One then becomes familiar with the appearance of the structures with this light.

The teeth are inspected for number, caries and type of occlusion. The number of teeth present is compared with the averages for the age. Occasionally a tooth will be seen in the newborn. Delayed appearance of the deciduous teeth, i.e., after one year of age, may be normal especially in obese children, or may indicate cretinism, rickets, congenital syphilis or mongolism. Absence of teeth is seen with congenital ectodermal dysplasia. Loss of teeth is seen in children with such metabolic diseases as acrodynia, xanthomatosis or low-phosphatase rickets.

Flattened edges of the teeth are usually seen in children who grind their teeth. The usual causes of tooth grinding are psychological difficulties, mental deficiency, tiredness or local irritation.

Malocclusion may occur without obvious cause or after premature loss or prolonged retention of deciduous teeth, as a family characteristic, or in children with mouth-breathing, cleft palate, micrognathia or prognathism. One cause of malocclusion of permanent teeth is persistent thumbsucking after six years.

Dental caries, due to bacterial decay and disintegration of tooth substance, is difficult to detect without special instruments until cavitation occurs. Disintegration of the enamel may be detected with a sharp instrument, especially if tooth pain is present.

Poor tooth formation may be seen with systemic diseases such as hypocalcemia, congenital lues, hypoparathyroidism, severe infections and nutritional disturbances, including rickets. Defective enamel formation in primary teeth occurs in children with prenatally caused neurological defects. Green or black teeth may be found after iron ingestion or after death of the tooth; green teeth are also seen in children who had severe jaundice at birth. Red teeth are sometimes seen in those with porphyria. Brown teeth may be due to congenital defect in tooth formation. Mottled, pitted teeth may be seen following excess fluoride ingestion, and for some years after receiving tetracycline. Centrally notched, peg-shaped (Hutchinson's) permanent teeth may occur in children with congenital syphilis. Mulberry-like six-year molars occur in normal children but may also indicate congenital syphilis.

Salivation is noted. There is usually little salivary secretion until three months of age. Absence of salivation may indicate dehydration, fever, Mikulicz's syndrome, atropine ingestion or congenital ectodermal dysplasia. Drooling is normal until two years of age. Excessive salivation is seen in children normally with teething or with caries, infections of the mouth, mental deficiency, mercury poisoning, gingivostomatitis, acrodynia or infections of the salivary glands. Thick mucoid secretions are frequently noted following tracheal irritation. In the newborn, unswallowed saliva or excess mucoid secretions are noted with tracheoesophageal fistula, probably due to aspirated gastric secretions with secondary tracheal irritation. Collection of saliva in the mouth due to swallowing difficulty is noted in children with ninth or tenth cranial nerve injury, especially that due to poliomyelitis, diphtheria or myasthenia.

The child should be told that examination of the throat is not really painful, but may be uncomfortable, and that the examination will take "only a second."

Further examination requires now that the mouth be opened farther and the jaws separated. At this point in the examination the child is raised to a sitting position (Fig. 15). If the child is eighteen months or older, it is worth while to try to get him to open his mouth voluntarily. One device is to ask if he would like to examine a relative (brother, sister, cousin). Most children say "Yes." Give him a tongue blade and say, "I'll show you how to do it. First you have your brother open his mouth wide Then you look at his teeth, then you look high, then you look low." Even though a gag is elicited, most children are not as angry as one would expect.

If suggestion fails, an attempt is made to place the tongue blade on the anterior part of the tongue for a view of the tongue and palate. With the blade in this position, the child is not uncomfortable and usually does not resist

Fig. 15. Restraint of patient in sitting position to examine posterior pharynx and epiglottis.

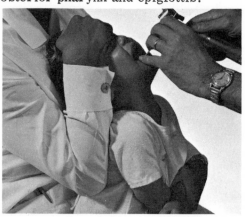

patient examination. If, however, the child resists, closes his mouth, and grits his teeth, he is carefully and firmly restrained.

Restraint can be maintained by asking the mother to hold the patient's hands and forehead. The tongue blade is then placed through the lips to the posterior teeth. Small tongue blades should be used for small children. Patiently, one pushes the blade between the teeth toward the pharynx. The blade should be inserted with a slightly downward motion so that the tongue is pushed forward and the base of the tongue downward. Suddenly, the child will gag, the mouth will open, and in this instant all the structures inside the mouth must be observed. At no time should the nose be pinched closed (see Fig. 15).

In order to grasp well what one sees, the examiner must develop the facility of anticipating the normal throat structures, and then retaining an after-image of the abnormalities seen. With practice, moreover, one learns to prolong the gag, so that the structures can be more carefully visualized. Older children are asked to breathe in and out through the mouth and careful note is made of all the oral structures which can be seen. If a large portion of the posterior nasopharynx cannot be observed, a tongue depressor is then introduced, the patient is told to say "aaah" or to breathe rapidly through the mouth, and gagging can usually be avoided. Frequently, if the patient sticks his tongue out and breathes deeply, the tongue blade is unnecessary.

Inflammation, color, swelling, and distortions of the gums and gingiva are noted. Redness, swelling and tenderness of the gums are noted in children with gingivitis. Inflammation of the gingiva may indicate the presence of a systemic disease or vitamin C deficiency, or may occur in mouth breathers or in children with erupting teeth, poor mouth hygiene, or poor dental care.

In a child with teeth, a black line along the margin of the gum may signify heavy metal poisoning. However, a melanotic line of the gums themselves is found in normal Negro infants. The gums near the teeth are purple and bleed easily in children with scurvy. The gums may also bleed easily in children with other bleeding diseases such as leukemia or chronic leukopenia, poor oral hygiene and, sometimes, in apparently normal children. The gums in children with herpetic stomatitis appear to be painted with a bright red pencil and are swollen and tender. Generalized hypertrophy of the gums is seen in mouth breathers, in children receiving dilantin with dilantin sensitivity, in children with hereditary gingival fibromatosis, and with many vitamin-deficiency states. Pin-point <u>inflamed</u> <u>elevations</u> from which pus can be expressed with the tongue depressor are characteristic of root abscess of the tooth.

In the young infant, epithelial pearls or <u>retention</u> <u>cysts</u> are found in or near the midline of the gums. These cysts have no clinical significance and usually disappear spontaneously at two or three months of age. White patches on the cheeks or lips in the older child which are asymptomatic may represent ectopic sebaceous glands, Fordyce's spots.

Next, the <u>buccal</u> <u>mucosa</u> is inspected. In the young infant one looks especially for thrush, small white patches which do not scrape off. Patches which scrape off are usually due to milk or other ingested white food. Other lesions of the buccal mucosa are described below. Bluish white scattered spots on the buccal mucosa at the level of the lower teeth and within the lower lip, each spot about the size of a grain of sand, are characteristic of <u>Koplik's</u> spots. These spots are pathognomonic of measles. Red spots 1-3 mm. in diameter over the buccal mucosa and palate are characteristic of Forschheimer's spots, frequently an early sign of German measles. Vesicles on the buccal mucosa, especially if surrounded by a red line, are usually due to herpes simplex. Similar vesicles, if found on the posterior pharynx, usually indicate herpangina due to Coxsackie infection. Pale red spots may cover the buccal mucosa in measles and other viral diseases, and are the <u>enanthems</u> of the diseases with skin exanthems. Other lesions seen on the buccal mucosa are described as they are seen further in the mouth.

<u>Veins</u> on the buccal mucosa are ordinarily not seen. Visible or dilated veins seen on the buccal mucosa or

tongue may be an early sign of cyanosis or may indicate cardiac failure or local vascular obstruction.

The tongue is inspected. Normally, the dorsal surface of the tongue is coated with conical filiform papillae; the reddish color is due to the blood supply to the papillae. Coating is significant only of lack of motion of the tongue due to debility in severe disease, or it may be due to mouth breathing. Dry tongue is a sign of general dehydration.

Tremor of the tongue is noted as it protrudes. Fine tremor is seen with chorea, hyperthyroidism or amyotonia congenita. Gross tremor may be seen in children with cerebral palsy. Fibrillations, slow undulating movements, indicate completely denervated muscle.

Large red papillae resembling a strawberry or raspberry are seen with scarlet fever. White spots of thrush may be noted in the newborn infant, when they are due to maternal infection, and also in debilitated children, in children with hypoparathyroidism, and following prolonged antibiotic medication. A triangular red area along the outer margin of the tongue occurs in patients with typhoid fever. A sore red tongue is seen with riboflavin or niacin deficiency states or with severe anemia. A uniformly smooth tongue with no apparent fungiform papillae is a sign of a hereditary disease, familial dysautonomia. Increased melanotic pigment of the buccal mucosa is seen in adrenal insufficiency and also in acanthosis nigricans, severe cachexia, neurofibromatosis, and pellagra. Occasionally melanotic patches are seen on the tongue of children with polyposis, Peutz's syndrome. Black tongue may be congenital, but has been described as a low-grade infection following penicillin administration or chickenpox. It also occurs in mouth bleeders, as in hemophilia.

Geographic tongue consists of gray, irregular areas of the tongue, and is usually due to unknown benign cause, but it may be related to febrile states or to allergy. It does not usually occur after six years of age. Deep furrows in the tongue are seen in mental defectives, particularly mongoloids, and are due to biting of the protruding tongue. Most commonly, however, furrowed tongue is a

congenital characteristic. <u>Scars</u> on the tongue may be due
to previous convulsions.

Macroglossia, or large tongue, is usually congenital.
It may be an early sign of hypothyroidism or gargoylism,
or be due to a lymphangioma, cyst or hemangioma. The
tongue may appear large in mongolism and other mental
defectives due to letting the tongue hang out. Protrusion
of the tongue may also be due to a tumor or thyroglossal
duct cyst at the base of the tongue.

<u>Tonguetie</u> is due to a very short frenum. If the
tongue tip of the infant does not interfere with feeding,
or if the older child can elevate the tip to produce the
sounds of t, d, n, or l, the condition does not exist. <u>Cysts</u>
or ranulae are occasionally seen in the floor of the mouth
near the frenum.

Paralysis of the tongue may be noted. The tongue
protrudes toward the involved side in patients with hypo-
glossal nerve lesions.

With the tongue depressor still on the anterior half
of the tongue, the hard <u>palate</u> is inspected. <u>Color</u> of the
palate is noted. Jaundice may easily be seen. <u>Petechiae</u>
on the palate are usually due to any condition causing
pharyngitis but may be due to other diseases which cause
petechiae on the skin or elsewhere.

Congenital <u>cleft</u> <u>palate</u> is easily observed. Note
should be made if the cleft involves only the hard palate,
the soft palate or the uvula and should be distinguished
from the rare condition of palatal perforation. <u>Perfora-
tion</u> of the palate is seen in children with congenital syphilis after they are two years of age. <u>High arched</u> palates
are usually seen in mouth breathers, but also in children
with arachnodactyly and many other disorders. Hypertrophy of the bone in the midline of the palate, torus
palatinus, is usually an anomaly of little significance.

The tongue depressor is then advanced over the root
of the tongue and pressed down. This usually causes
gagging and is an unpleasant part of the routine examination. Because the child almost immediately resists further manipulation, this part of the examination should be
done expeditiously, and the examiner should know exactly

what he wishes to learn before causing the child to gag.

The first area that presents with the gag is the epi-glottis, located at the base of the tongue. Swelling and color should be noted. A swollen red epiglottis is seen in some children with laryngotracheobronchitis, especially when it is due to H. influenzae, and may obstruct respira-tion. A swollen pale epiglottis is seen with viral infections or allergy and may represent a respiratory emergency. Congenitally large epiglottis or ulcers of the epiglottis may be noted.

The uvula is next inspected. A very long uvula is congenital and may cause gagging or coughing. Occasion-ally the uvula is congenitally bifid. It may be absent, having been accidentally removed during tonsillectomy. Motion of the uvula and soft palate are noted as the patient is gagged, or is told to say "aaah." Paralysis of the soft palate or uvula or absence of the gag reflex is an early sign of poliomyelitis or diphtheria, but it is seen also in other disorders involving the glossopharyngeal or vagus nerves, and with masses behind the palate. Limited motion of the soft palate may be caused by hypertrophied, infected adenoids. A translucent membrane in the mid-line of the soft palate indicates lack of continuity of mus-cles and may be a sign of palatopharyngeal incompetence.

The posterior pharynx is noted for lymphoid hyper-plasia, color, postnasal drip, membrane, edema, exudate, abscess or vesicles. Lymphoid hyperplasia is seen with any infection of the area. A red inflamed pharynx is characteristic of any type of acute pharyngitis, but there are not good local signs to distinguish bacterial from non-bacterial pharyngitis. A pale, puffy mucosa indicates edema. Vesicles on the posterior pharynx, anterior pillars or uvula surrounded by 3-6 mm. of erythema are a sign of herpangina due to Coxsackie A infection. These ulcerate, and small ulcers may remain for two or three weeks. Small maculopapules on the posterior pharynx also are seen in other respiratory viral diseases.

Profuse postnasal drip indicates infection in the nose, nasopharynx, or sinuses, and may cause a foul odor. A white membrane over the tonsils or posterior pharynx is seen in children with diphtheria, other bacterial infections, particularly Vincent's angina or beta-streptococcal infection, infectious mononucleosis, agranulocytosis, or leukemia. In diphtheria, the mouth smells "mousy" and the membrane pulls away with bleeding. The membrane in diphtheria is usually more confluent and spreads to cover more of the uvula and posterior pharynx than the other infections. Indeed, a confluent membrane involving the uvula or posterior pharynx should be considered diphtheritic until proved otherwise.

The pharynx or throat is separated from the mouth by the anterior and posterior pillars. The palatine (faucial) tonsils are located between these pillars. Size of the tonsils is noted. Tonsils, as all lymphoid tissue, are much larger during early childhood than later; therefore, statements regarding enlargement of tonsils in childhood must be reserved until many normal tonsils have been examined or unless obstruction of the airway is obvious.

Crypts in the tonsillar tissue may indicate past infection; pus in the tonsils and peritonsillar abscesses indicate acute infections. The tonsils appear to be pushed backward or forward and the uvula may be displaced with peritonsillar abscesses. Peritonsillar abscesses occur more often in older children and are usually due to streptococcus infections.

In the infant under two years of age erythema of the tonsils usually occurs with bacterial infections, especially streptococci, pneumococci, or H. influenzae, and purulent exudate or membrane suggests the presence of viral infections. In children over two years some attempt can be made to distinguish bacterial from viral tonsillitis, though most often it is necessary to obtain cultures of the nasopharynx. Yellow or grayish-white follicles are usually due to bacteria. Vesicles, nodules, punched-out ulcers, scanty or streaky membranes, or patchy gray, white or yellow membranes usually indicate viral infection. A coalescent white membrane occurs with Candida infections. A coalescent adherent membrane is common in diphtheria. A bluish-gray membrane with ulceration is more common in children with agranulocytosis or with other severe underlying hematological disorders.

Tuberculosis and tumors may also cause enlargement of the tonsils. Definite <u>unilateral</u> enlargement of the tonsillar area is common with such diseases as Vincent's infection, diphtheria and lymphoma. Enlarged, lobulated, red-orange tonsils have been reported in association with accumulation of cholesterol esters, Tangier disease.

Collections of movable mucus and pus may be noted in the posterior pharynx. This is usually postnasal drip and may be caused by sinusitis or infected adenoids.

Out-pouching of the posterior pharyngeal wall is characteristic of posterior pharyngeal abscess. Examination of the retropharynx with a finger is usually necessary only if a retropharyngeal abscess is suspected. Retropharyngeal abscesses usually occur in the first two years of life; they are felt as unilateral soft masses in infants who are usually quite ill, with noisy respirations and, occasionally, retracted necks.

Single ulcers without generalized symptoms are "canker sores." A recurrent type of canker sore may occur with allergy. Sudden swelling of any part of the buccal mucosa also occurs with allergy.

Other types of stomatitis occurring on the mucosa include vesicles of chickenpox, mucous patches of early congenital syphilis and general inflammation with vesicles of the erythroderma desquamativum syndromes.

<u>Vomiting</u> is really a symptom. However, when vomiting is seen the nature of the vomitus should be noted and the vomitus saved if physical and chemical examinations are desired. Vomiting in the newborn may have special significance and is described later.

Overfeeding, food intolerance and improper handling of the child are the usual causes of vomiting during infancy. However, vomiting of recently ingested food may be an early sign of infection in the intestinal tract or elsewhere in children. Other common causes of "nondescript" vomiting include severe coughing, brain tumor and increased intracranial pressure, psychogenic factors, food allergy, chalasia, poisoning including lead poisoning and, perhaps, abdominal epilepsy. A common form of severe vomiting is seen in children two to twelve years of age; it occurs periodically, is probably due to a combination of psychogenic factors and lability of ketone-producing mechanisms and is termed "cyclic vomiting." Vomiting with nausea before breakfast may indicate hypoglycemia. Vomiting without nausea, especially in the early morning, may be a sign of brain tumor.

Forceful vomiting in the infant, especially of curdled milk free of bile-staining, may be a sign of pylorospasm or pyloric stenosis. Vomitus containing bile may indicate duodenal or jejunal obstruction, whereas fecal vomiting is seen more commonly in children with lower intestinal obstruction, ileus or peritonitis.

Bloody vomitus is most commonly due to swallowed blood from the nose and upper respiratory tract or from the mother's fissured nipple in a breast-fed infant. It is also seen in children with hemorrhagic diseases including Henoch-Schoenlein purpura, following the ingestion of foreign body or poisons, or following severe vomiting from any cause. Occasionally, bloody vomitus is seen in children with gastric, duodenal or esophageal ulcers, and in children with anomalies of the portal vein or with cirrhosis of the liver with esophageal varices.

LARYNX

The voice is noted for hoarseness or stridor, which may easily be determined from the cry of the infant or the voice of the child. Either of these may indicate respiratory tract obstruction. In the newborn, hoarseness or stridor is characteristic of hypocalcemia, congenital laryngeal or epiglottic anomalies, laryngeal tumor, thyroglossal duct cyst, or injury to the laryngeal nerve. In infancy hoarseness or stridor may also be due to a vascular ring surrounding the trachea, hypothyroidism, laryngeal infections or laryngotracheobronchitis. In addition to those causes already mentioned, in the older child hoarseness may result from shouting, laryngitis (including laryngitis due to diphtheria or measles), bulbar poliomyelitis, tetanus, Gaucher's disease, retropharyngeal abscess, foreign body, allergy or croup. Unless good presumptive cause of the hoarseness exists, laryngoscopy is necessary. Hoarseness due to infection is more commonly found in viral laryngitis or laryngitis due to H. influenzae than in that due to streptococci. A low raucous cry is found in cretins; a growl, in deLange's syndrome. A sharp whining cry is found in infants with severe gastrointestinal disturbances such as intussusception or peritonitis. A cat-like cry is heard in some children with a rare chromosome abnormality. Nasal speech may occur in children with chronic upper respiratory infection, enlarged adenoids, deafness or neurogenic or anatomic velopharyngeal incompetence such as that seen with cleft palate.

Laryngoscopy is not performed in the routine examination. If indicated, it is best performed in the small child with an electric laryngoscope of small or medium size with good batteries and light. The child should have an empty stomach to obviate aspiration of vomitus during manipulation, and he is placed in a supine position. The head is held with the neck partly flexed by the mother. The child's tongue is held and the laryngoscope is slowly inserted along the tongue to the base.

The posterior pharynx and epiglottis are visualized and their status noted. A redundant large epiglottis may be seen when it obstructs the airway.

The laryngoscope is then passed over the epiglottis and the handle pulled up slightly toward the patient's head until the larynx is visualized. Laryngeal spasm, edema, paralysis, stenosis, redundancy or tumors may be noted. Thyroglossal duct cysts at the base of the tongue may be seen. The subglottic area is also seen if the larynx itself is normal.

In the older child who can cooperate, indirect laryngoscopy is less traumatic. The patient is seated, the mirror warmed, the tongue grasped, and the mirror then passed back to rest on the anterior surface of the uvula, pushing it upward and backward. With good lighting, the larynx is visualized. The cords are best seen if the patient is told to say "Eeee." This is the best diagnostic method for examination of the larynx when it can be used. It is particularly useful in problems of laryngeal motility and should always precede direct laryngoscopy if possible.

In the older child specific speech defects such as lisping or stuttering should be noted. Deep voices occur in adolescent males and in children with adrenogenital syndrome or with sexual precocity of other types. A nasal voice is heard in children with large adenoids, sinusitis or palatal paralysis. Delayed or limited speech occurs in children who are deaf or mentally retarded or who have neurological or physical abnormalities of the vocalizing apparatus. The child should speak a word or two at ten months to one year, and have the ability to put two or three words together to make a sentence by two years. Slurred indistinct speech with clicking produced by the tongue forcibly hitting the hard palate occurs in chorea. Aphonia with ability to whisper may indicate hysteria.

NECK

The examination of the neck takes one or two seconds but may help in the diagnosis of many diseases. The patient should be lying flat on his back.

First, the size of the neck is noted. The neck normally appears short during infancy and lengthens at about three or four years of age. A short neck is also seen in children with platybasia, Morquio's disease, cretinism, gargoylism, and the Klippel-Feil syndrome. Webbing of the neck is sometimes noted in children with gonadal dysgenesis, or as an isolated anomaly. Marked edema of the neck is noted in children with diphtheria, local infections, cellulitis, other infections of the mouth, mumps and any of the causes of generalized edema.

Next, one palpates the anterior and posterior cervical triangles for lymph nodes. In general, their significance is described in Chapter III.

Cervical nodes more than 1 cm. in diameter are enlarged. They drain the sinuses, ears, mouth, teeth and pharynx.

Other masses in the neck are observed or palpated.
Enlarged parotids usually extend down into the neck. Cystic
masses in the midline high in the neck which are freely
movable and move upward when the patient swallows may
be thyroglossal duct cysts. Pulling the tongue forward
causes such cystic areas to move. Fistula may accompany
the cyst. Midline cyst-like masses which do not move
freely may be dermoids. Diffuse swelling of the neck with
non-pitting edema - "bull neck" - is seen in children with
severe diphtheria.

The sternocleidomastoid muscle is then palpated. A
mass in the lower third of the sternocleidomastoid muscle
generally indicates congenital torticollis. Oval, cystic,
smooth, moderately movable masses near the upper third
of the muscle are usually due to branchial cysts and may
be associated with fistula or may be attached to the skin
with a small dimple. These are almost always anterior
to the sternocleidomastoid muscle.

Next, one palpates the trachea, feeling first the most
anterior parts with one finger and then going down both
sides simultaneously with the thumb and index finger. The
trachea should be slightly to the right of the midline. Any
further deviation in either direction indicates mediastinal
shift due to atelectasis (especially due to foreign body),
effusion, pneumothorax or tumor in the chest or neck.

A palpatory thud (or audible slap) may be felt or
heard over the trachea and may indicate the presence of
a foreign body free in the trachea.

Then, one feels just below the thyroid cartilage for
the thyroid isthmus, and both lobes of the thyroid just
lateral to the thyroid cartilage. The thyroid in the younger
child can be felt with the child supine, and the thumb on
one side and the index and second fingers on the opposite
side of the thyroid cartilage. In the older child, it may
be easier to palpate the thyroid from behind with two fingers of each hand on both sides of the thyroid cartilage.
The thyroid is observed or felt to move upward when the
patient swallows. Size, shape, position, mobility and
tenderness are noted.

Thyroid enlargement may be due to hyperactive

thyroid, malignancy or goiter. A smooth enlarged thyroid
mass indicates thyroid hyperplasia. Nodules in the thyroid
are usually adenomatous and may be malignant. Enlarged
tender thyroid indicates early thyroiditis. A woody feel is
characteristic of Hashimoto's thyroiditis. Bruit over the
thyroid is common with thyroid enlargement.

Goiter with hypothyroidism may be due to antithyroid
drugs or foods, Hashimoto's thyroiditis, enzymatic defect
in hormone synthesis, or a deficit in iodine. Hypothyroidism without goiter may be hereditary, congenital or familial,
or may be due to pituitary disease, sarcoid or xanthomatosis.

The area just above either clavicle is observed and
palpated. An ill-defined soft mass which changes in size
with crying or respiration in the infant is most commonly
a cystic hygroma arising from the mediastinum. This
mass can usually be transilluminated. A hard mass may
be the callus of a fractured clavicle; a palpable node in
this area may be the first enlarged node of Hodgkin's
disease.

The vessels of the neck are observed. Enlarged
veins or abnormal venous pulsations may be due to increased venous pressure which may be caused by heart
failure, pericarditis, or masses in the mediastinum.
Pulsation of the carotids may sometimes be seen in children, usually after exercise or emotional upset, but may
indicate aortic insufficiency. Venous pulsations in the
neck in the upright child are always abnormal. Venous
pulsations, in contrast to arterial pulsation, are obliterated by light jugular compression. Distended neck
veins do not occur in patients with severe liver disease
unless heart disease is also present. When heart failure
is suspected, press on the liver. If the jugular veins become prominent, failure is present. This is the hepato-
jugular reflex, but is not a good sign in the very young
because they perform a Valsalva maneuver on abdominal
pressure, making the jugular veins stand out. If the
jugular veins do not fill on liver pressure, the venous
system is not patent. This is a sign of hepatic vein
thrombosis (Budd-Chiari syndrome).

Venous pressure can be fairly accurately determined

by measuring the distance from the upper border of the
clavicle to the upper level of venous distention in the neck
with the child in the sitting position.

The carotid sinus may be massaged in those children
who have histories indicative of possible heart block. This
is done only with the stethoscope on the chest. The carotid
sinus is best reached by following the carotid artery up to
the angle of the jaw and covering the whole area with the
thumb. Massage of this area, one side at a time, normally slows the heart 10-20 beats per minute. A greater
decrease in rate indicates abnormal carotid sensitivity,
a rare cause of syncope.

The neck should be auscultated with the bell stethoscope. Murmurs may be heard particularly over the
carotid area, but also elsewhere in the neck, and are frequently transmitted from the heart with organic disease.
To and fro bruits may be heard over an enlarged thyroid.
Other sounds in the neck may indicate other vascular
anomalies such as those seen with cerebrovascular insufficiency. Bruits from aortic stenosis murmurs are heard
bilaterally low in the middle part of the neck or at the
angles of the jaw, the carotid areas. Those of vascular
insufficiency are usually unilateral. Transmitted sounds
from the trachea may obliterate these sounds, except
during the clear interval between inspiration and expiration.

Finally, motion of the neck is noted, first by asking
the patient to touch his chest with his chin and to turn his
head from side to side. If he is unable to do this the examiner raises the patient's head from the pillow with one
hand and then turns the patient's head from side to side.
Resistance to flexion of the neck, stiff neck, is characteristic of meningitis or meningeal irritation; in debilitated children with these diseases, the neck may remain
supple.

Stiff neck may also be noted with the viral encephalitides, tetanus, lead poisoning, meningismus and rheumatoid arthritis. It is noted with pharyngitis, cervical
adenitis, retropharyngeal abscess, subluxation of the cervical vertebrae due to retropharyngeal or peritonsillar abscess, herniation of the cerebellar tonsils with increased

intracranial pressure, and with degenerative nervous
system diseases as part of their generalized hypertonia.
Hyperextension of the neck, opisthotonos, is due to any
of the causes of stiff neck of a more severe degree and
is also seen in children with cerebral palsy or kernicterus.   Brudzinski's sign, obtained by flexing the neck
and noting flexion at the hip, knee or ankle, is a similar
indication of central nervous system irritation.

The tonic neck reflex is obtained by placing the patient on his back and turning his head to one side.   The
ipsilateral arm and leg flex and the contralateral arm and
leg extend.   The head is turned to the opposite side and
the position of the limbs reverses.   In practice, the opposite flexion and extension may occur and still the test
be positive.   This reflex is present at birth and lasts
three to five months normally.   If present after this time,
brain damage should be suspected.

Inability to move the neck from side to side may accompany any of the above states and is seen also with congenital torticollis, the Klippel-Feil syndrome and occasionally cervical rib.   Neurological torticollis occurs in patients with lesions of the spinal accessory nerve, causing
sternocleidomastoid and trapezius muscle paralysis; or
without apparent cause.   Eye lesions, especially when
vision is unequal, or labyrinthitis, spasmus nutans or
brain tumors may be accompanied by torticollis.   If the
patient cannot maintain his head elevated, head drop,
early poliomyelitis or other muscle weakness should be
considered.

Voluntary tilting of the neck may be seen in children
with habit spasm, brain tumors, poor vision or strabismus.   Head-tilting from side to side may occur in children
in whom the corpus callosum is absent.   Head rolling and
nodding may be due to habit spasm, mental retardation,
eye or ear abnormalities or chorea.

CHAPTER V

The Chest

Many disease states can be diagnosed by simply looking at the chest. This fact is helpful, since sometimes it is difficult to do more than observe the hyperactive or crying patient. The order of examination of the chest in a child depends on the attitude of the child; some find it easier to listen to the chest first, before the child starts to cry, and then to proceed with the other parts of the examination, while others observe and palpate first and use the stethoscope later.

INSPECTION

The general shape and circumference of the chest are noted. The chest circumference is obtained at the nipple line. It is normally the same as or slightly less than the head circumference for the first two years of life and then exceeds the head circumference. In very sturdy children, the chest circumference is slightly greater than that of the head even during the first two years. Marked disproportion between head and chest measurements requires comparison with standards for the child's age. Disproportions are usually due to abnormal head growth rather than abnormal chest growth. When the measurements are compared with standards, however, the part causing abnormal growth can usually be determined.

In the premature infant, the rib cage is thin and the chest may collapse with every inspiration. In infancy the chest is almost round, the anteroposterior diameter equaling the transverse diameter. As the child grows older, the chest normally expands in the transverse di-

ameter. A round or emphysematous chest in the child after the age of six years suggests a chronic pulmonary disease such as asthma. A funnel-shaped chest, characterized by sternal depression, may be a congenital anomaly
or may indicate adenoid hypertrophy. A short wide chest
is noted especially in short children or in children with
Morquio's disease. Pigeon breast, in which the sternum
protrudes, is noted as an isolated anomaly or in children
with rickets or osteopetrosis. The xiphisternum may
protrude and appear broken, but this condition is normal
in the young child and is due only to a loose attachment between the xiphoid and the body of the sternum. As in adults,
note is made of the rib numbers to orient the examiner.
The second rib attaches at the angle of the sternum just
below the clavicles.

With the patient on his back, swellings at the costo-
chondral junction may be seen. These swellings or blunt
knobbings form the rachitic rosary. Almost always a depression will be noted in the child in the region of the 8th
to 10th ribs and the bottom of the rib cage will appear to
flare. The depression at the site of the diaphragm muscle
leaving the chest wall is known as Harrison's groove.
Unless the flaring is marked, it is not diagnostic of any
disease. Although it occurs in rickets, this type of flaring is also found in many children with any pulmonary
disorder, in children who were born prematurely and in
many normal young children who have no obvious patho-
logic disturbance.

The angle made by the lower rib margin with the
sternum is noted. Ordinarily, this angle is about 45 degrees. A larger angle may be found in children with lung
disease and a smaller angle in those with malnutrition and
deficiency states. Note is made of expansion of the chest.
Most of a child's normal respiratory activity is effected
by abdominal motion until age six or seven years, and
there is very little intercostal motion. Later, thoracic
motion becomes responsible for air exchange. If the interspaces show much motion, lung disease or peritonitis is
suggested. One should note whether the motion of the
interspaces is restricted to one side. There is less motion on the involved side with pneumonia, hydro- or pneumo-

thorax, obstructive foreign body or atelectasis, and increased motion on the opposite side of the chest in these
states. These disease states and paralysis of the chest
musculature also produce increased motion of the diaphragm. With normal respiration, the chest expands, the
sternal angle increases and the diaphragm descends on
inspiration; the reverse occurs with expiration. Paradoxical respiration is noted when the diaphragm appears
to rise on inspiration and to descend on expiration. Paradoxical motion of the chest and diaphragm may be produced
by any of the disease states mentioned, particularly pneumothorax. That side of the chest which is involved tends to
collapse on inspiration and remains stationary or appears
to expand on expiration. Paradoxical respiration is also
noted in children with neuromuscular diseases such as
phrenic nerve paralysis, poliomyelitis, or chorea.

One can sometimes tell the difference between high
obstruction and low obstruction. Retraction is chiefly
suprasternal and severe in high obstruction, such as
laryngeal lesions, but mainly infrasternal in low obstruction, such as infantile bronchiolitis. Retractions are
usually less intense in lower obstruction. Diseases like
croup, congenital laryngeal stridor, stridor due to injury
of the laryngeal nerves, diphtheria, bronchiolitis and
diseases of the abdomen such as peritonitis, and also
paralysis of the diaphragm produce marked retraction
above and below the sternum with marked intercostal
activity bilaterally.

It is important to note asymmetry. Precordial
bulging may be diagnostic of an inter-atrial septal defect,
other causes of right ventricular enlargement, pneumothorax, or a chronic localized chest disease. Lung tumors such as Ewing's sarcoma involving the lung may
cause asymmetry, as may congenital absence of the
chest muscles. Asymmetry is, however, most commonly
found secondary to scoliosis.

The position of the scapulae is noted for anomalies
such as Sprengel's deformity, winged scapula, and Klippel-
Feil syndrome, which are described with the examination
of the spine (Chapter VII).

BREASTS

Breast development is noted.

It is usually difficult to determine whether a breast which appears large is simply hypertrophic or is truly developmentally enlarged. The simple hypertrophic breast usually has a flat nipple with a small areola, and the breast tissue feels soft. The developed breast usually has protrusion of the nipple, enlargement of the areola and a firmness to the tissue underlying the areola. Redness, heat and tenderness around the breast may indicate infection, mastitis. Unless there is some unusual question about the breast or its development, the breasts of both boys and girls ordinarily should be inspected but not palpated. Ordinarily, the neonatal breast is enlarged for about one or two months. In girls, normal breast development begins about the 10th to 14th year of age. One breast usually begins to develop before the other and is frequently tender. Precocious breast development in girls is usually normal but of unknown cause. Other causes of precocious breast development include stilbestrol ingestion, ovarian tumors or precocity from any cause. Pseudoprecocious breast enlargement occurs in fat children and is due merely to adipose tissue. Small round hard nodules in the breasts of children, as in adults, may be due to cysts or tumors; these masses are usually non-tender, are usually irregular, and may feel attached to the skin or grow out of proportion to the remainder of the breast tissue.

True gynecomastia in boys is usually due to unknown benign factors at puberty but may be due to tumors of the breast, severe liver disease and, very rarely, gonadal or adrenal lesions. Usually, breast enlargement in the male is due only to adipose tissue, but it may occur with gonadal dysgenesis, Klinefelter's syndrome. Gynecomastia may occur with digitalis administration.

Breast development is absent in adolescent girls with pituitary failure, anorexia nervosa starting before puberty, gonadal dysgenesis, adrenal hyperplasia or severe malnutrition.

LUNGS

The type and rate of breathing are next noted. A newborn child, especially the premature, will normally have Cheyne-Stokes type of breathing, characterized by periods of deep and rapid respirations alternating with periods of slow, shallow respirations or no respiratory activity, apnea; this should disappear by four weeks of life when breathing becomes regular. Various brain or metabolic lesions which depress the central respiratory center may cause Cheyne-Stokes respirations.

The rate of respiration varies from 30-50 at birth, 16-20 at six years of age, and 14-16 at puberty. Young children tend to have an abnormally high respiratory rate with even slight excitement, so that estimation of true respiratory rate is best obtained when the infant or young child is asleep. A rapid respiratory rate, tachypnea, is found almost always in children with any type of respiratory disorder, and a normal rate usually indicates lack of acute pulmonary disease. Children below the age of three years with upper airway obstruction rarely breathe faster than 50 per minute, while those with lower airway obstructive disease such as bronchiolitis frequently breathe at rates of 80-100. In young children, tachypnea may be an early sign of heart failure.

A rapid respiratory rate also occurs frequently in children with generalized or localized infection, fever, poisoning, salicylism, acidosis or shock. A slow rate suggests central respiratory depression, especially that due to increased intracranial pressure, sedatives or other drugs, alkalosis or poisons. Slow jerky respiratory movements or bursts of hyperpnea alternating with apnea, Biot's breathing, may be seen with central nervous system lesions involving the respiratory center such as encephalitis or bulbar poliomyelitis.

The depth of respiration is noted. Deep respirations are termed hyperpnea. Depth of respiration is an indication of the degree of anoxia present, the state of activity of the respiratory center and the presence of acidosis or alkalosis.

In obstructive respiratory diseases, breathing will

usually be rapid and may be deep or shallow, depending
on the degree and nature of the obstruction. In metabolic
acidosis, breathing is deep and the respiratory rate is
usually rapid. In early metabolic alkalosis, breathing is
deep and the rate is rapid. Respiration is depressed in
alkalosis of long duration. Listening with the bell of the
stethoscope over the mouth of a small child helps in estimating the rate and depth of respiration and frequently
assists in diagnosing the degree of acidosis.

It is worthwhile to establish one's own standards for
depth of respiration of children. This is easily done if a
group of children aged one, three, six, nine and twelve
months, one, two, three, four, five, six, eight and ten
years are studied. The children are examined in their
normal posture and also lying down. During normal respiration, air from the child's nose will be felt a measurable
distance from the nose. This is recorded for each age.
This figure, plus or minus one inch, is then a measurement of the normal for each examiner. The author's measurements for the above ages, when the patients are supine,
are 2 and 3 inches for infants one and three months of age
respectively; 4 inches for six, nine and 12 months; 5 and
6 inches for one and two years of age respectively; 8 inches
for 3 and 4 years of age; 9 inches for 5 and 6 years of age;
and 10 inches for 8 and 10 years of age. Increased depth
of respiration is indicated by feeling the breath farther
away, and decreased, closer to the nose.

Dyspnea, or distress during breathing, may be recognized by observing flaring of the nares and intercostal
spaces, cyanosis, supra- and infrasternal retraction and
rapid respiratory rate. One should try to note whether the
distress is mainly inspiratory or expiratory; inspiratory
distress occurs more frequently with high obstructions and
expiratory with low obstructions. Dyspnea may also occur
with exercise, pain, fright, anemia, cardiovascular disorders, hyperthyroidism and many other conditions.

Dyspnea is usually increased by exercise. This fact
forms the basis of the exercise tolerance test. If limitation of exercising ability is suspected, some type of graded
measurement of this ability is desirable. Usually, chil-

dren of various ages can be asked to run about or up and down stairs, and are then compared with their peers for the development of dyspnea. Dyspnea which occurs too soon indicates any state which may cause anoxia, or such causes as lack of habit of exercise, obesity or emotional distress. Exercise of the arms causes more dyspnea than an equivalent amount of exercise of the lower extremities.

Cough is noted. Cough may be due to laryngeal or pulmonary infection, postnasal drip, pulmonary anomalies, chronic pulmonary disease, foreign body in the esophagus or respiratory tract, cardiac failure, allergy, emotion, habit or extrinsic masses, including vascular ring around the trachea. Expiratory paroxysmal cough followed by an inspiratory whoop in a child over six months of age, or followed by vomiting in a child less than six months of age, is characteristic of pertussis, parapertussis, and respiratory infection following pertussis. A loose productive cough is noted in those with bronchitis, upper respiratory infection with postnasal drip and cystic fibrosis of the pancreas with pulmonary involvement. A sharp, brassy, nonproductive, barking cough is heard in children with laryngeal diphtheria, foreign body, croup and, occasionally, tuberculosis. A tight nonproductive cough is heard in the pneumonias.

Cough is usually non-productive in children, even with tuberculosis or bronchiectasis, and expectoration is rare. Hemoptysis may indicate foreign body, tuberculosis, other pulmonary infections, heart disease or bleeding from high in the respiratory tract; and purulent sputum may occur in children with chronic pulmonary disease. A dry, irritative, persistent cough is heard in children with measles, tracheitis or laryngitis.

The cough reflex can usually be elicited by causing the child to gag, examining the throat or, if necessary, blowing cigarette smoke near the child. The cough reflex may be depressed in children with mental retardation, debilitating disease, paralysis of the respiratory musculature, or in children who have received sedatives or cough depressants.

Palpation. -- <u>Palpation</u> is performed in children by placing the palm of the hand lightly but firmly on the chest and feeling with the palm and fingertips. The entire chest is palpated. Palpation is used to confirm one's observation of the chest wall, such as position of scapulae, asymmetry of chest, presence of rosary, Harrison's groove, position or fracture of clavicles, presence of breast tissue and presence of axillary lymph nodes. Any <u>masses</u> or areas of <u>tenderness</u> are noted. A <u>thud</u> is occasionally palpated high on the chest as the patient breathes. This is a sign of foreign body in the trachea. Palpation of the heart will be discussed below.

<u>Tactile fremitus</u> is easily determined by palpating the chest wall in children who are crying, or in children who can cooperate by speaking or who can be asked their name. Fremitus, when obtainable, is usually felt over the entire chest as a tingling sensation. Decrease in vocal fremitus suggests the presence of airway obstruction or may indicate pleural effusion. Fremitus when the patient does not make vocal sounds is normally absent, but it is frequently felt in children who have been crying and signifies a partial movable obstruction to the passage of air. Tactile fremitus is especially valuable in distinguishing the presence of mucus high in the respiratory tract, where fremitus is very coarse, from lower respiratory tract infection, where it is absent. Fremitus is a poor sign for distinguishing pneumonia, atelectasis or space-taking lesions in childhood.

One should palpate the <u>rib interspaces</u> for <u>retraction or paralysis</u> of the intercostal muscles. Excess motion of the interspaces is an indication of increased respiratory activity. Decreased motion of the interspaces may indicate paralysis of the intercostal muscles, decreased respiratory activity or, if unilateral, any of the causes of decreased respiration of one side of the chest. <u>Pulsation of the rib vessels</u> due to coarctation of the aorta almost never occurs in childhood. Pericardial or pleural <u>friction rubs</u> can occasionally be palpated and feel like fine vibrations.

The <u>axillary lymph</u> nodes are palpated best by bringing the palm of the hand flat into the axilla with the patient's

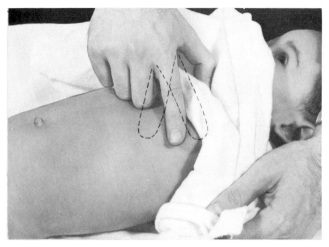

Fig. 16. Direct percussion.

arm hanging freely at his side. Slight rubbing motion will
indicate the size of the glands. Normally, several glands
up to 3 mm. in diameter will be felt in all children. Abnormalities of these nodes have been described in the section on Lymph Nodes (Chapter III).

Percussion. -- In percussing the chest, both direct
and indirect methods are used. In the direct (Fig. 16)
method the chest wall is tapped lightly with either the index or the middle finger. With this method every half-
inch of the chest is percussed quickly. This method is
rapid, gentle and informative but requires considerable
practice.

When the indirect method of percussion is used, a
finger of one hand is placed firmly on the chest wall, the
index or middle finger of the other hand is used as the
percussing hammer, and the same areas are covered.
The bases for good indirect percussion are: (1) the non-
percussing finger must be pressed firmly against the chest
wall; (2) no other fingers should touch the chest wall;
(3) the patient should be either sitting or standing, or else
lying flat on his back or abdomen; and (4) the percussing

finger should move like a piano hammer with a very loose hinge-joint action at the wrist. Because the chest wall is thinner and the muscles smaller, the chest seems more resonant in children than in adults. Therefore, it is much easier to get accurate information by examining the chest of a child than of an adult. If one percusses too vigorously, however, vibrations over a large area may obscure localized areas of dullness.

Posteriorly, one percusses from the shoulders down to dullness at the level of the eighth to tenth ribs, where the diaphragm causes a change in the note. It is important that the head be in the midline facing directly forward during this part of the examination. If the neck is twisted, aeration is not equal, and spurious dullness may be detected. The top of the diaphragm will usually be located at about the level of the apex of the costovertebral angle. Anteriorly, tapping is performed from just below the clavicle to the level of dullness. The sides of the chest are percussed from the axillae downward. Then, starting at the lower margin of the lung fields posteriorly and the upper abdomen anteriorly, the lower margins and the mobility of the diaphragm are determined. It is generally useful to percuss beginning in those areas where one expects resonance to where dullness is expected. This is especially important over the area of the heart.

A decreased percussion note, or dullness, will be found over the scapulae, the diaphragm, the liver and the heart. These areas should be well demarcated. Normally, the top of the liver is percussed anteriorly at about the level of the sixth rib from the midaxillary line to the sternum. The lower edge of the lung or the top of the diaphragm is usually percussed to the level of the eighth to tenth ribs posteriorly on both sides. Anteriorly, the diaphragm usually cannot be percussed below the level of the liver on the right. Occasionally, a distended stomach will cause hyperresonance on the left, so that one may have difficulty delineating the level of the diaphragm. Fortunately, most children have an indentation of the ribs at the attachment of the diaphragm to help indicate where dullness is expected. Usually, the diaphragm is percussed

anteriorly also at the level of the eighth to the tenth rib.
In all these areas, the diaphragm will usually be found to
move, as determined by changing dullness, one to two rib
spaces between inspiration and expiration. In the child
under two years of age, this motion is very difficult to
determine by percussion.

These normal areas of percussion dullness may be
altered as follows: liver dullness may be at a higher level
than the sixth rib in conditions causing liver enlargement
or elevation of the liver as in abdominal distention; or with
atelectasis of the lobes of the right lung. The liver will
be percussed at the level of the sixth rib on the left in
dextrocardia with levorotation of the liver or with situs
inversus. The diaphragm will be higher than normal in
conditions causing collapse of the lungs or distention of
the abdomen, and will be lower than normal in conditions
causing emphysema of the lungs with masses or space-
taking lesions in the chest.

The mediastinum in children is usually percussed
as the area of cardiac dullness. On rare occasions, a
broadened area of dullness above or at the level of the
base of the heart may be due to the thymus. Though this
is without significance, any broadening of the mediastinum
must be noted, as it may be due to presence of other
masses. Heart size will be altered by conditions altering
the heart, and are described below; as are conditions
causing a shift in the dullness of the heart or mediastinum.
Localized areas of decreased resonance, dullness or flat-
ness may be found in children with consolidation of the
lung, such as pneumonia; with lung collapse, atelectasis;
with increased fluid in the lung, as pulmonary edema; or
with accumulation of fluid in the pleural space, such as
pleural effusion or empyema. Very rarely, dull areas in
the chest may be due to the presence of tumors. Dullness
below the angle of the left scapula may occur with pericardial effusion (Ewart's or Pins's sign).

Hyperresonance of the chest is due to an increase in
the amount of air in the chest. It is found most commonly
in children with emphysema and is usually accompanied by
a lowered diaphragm. Localized hyperresonance may also

indicate the presence of free air in the chest, as occurs with pneumothorax; with loculated air as with lung cyst or abscess; obstructive foreign body, or diaphragmatic hernia. Increase in resonance over the area of the liver may indicate the presence of a ruptured abdominal viscus.

Auscultation. -- One listens then for breath sounds, rales, rhonchi and extraneous sounds. Especially during auscultation should the child be totally flat or totally erect as even slight turning of the head to one side may so decrease the breath sounds as to suggest severe pathological states. Because of the small size of the patient's chest, and because of the desire to localize pathological findings, the small bell stethoscope is most satisfactory for the usual auscultation in children. The inside of the stethoscope should be clean, the tubing intact and well-fitting and about 18 inches long. The stethoscope should be warmed before use and it must be pressed firmly against the chest wall or sounds which are artifacts will be heard. It is usually easier to get a tight fit of the stethoscope with the chest if the bell is placed in the interspaces rather than over the ribs. The entire chest, including the axillary areas, should be auscultated. Children's fingers must sometimes be restrained from touching the tubing during this part of the examination, as touching the tubing also makes extraneous sounds. It should be noted that if the stethoscope is not firmly on the chest, nothing will be heard!

Because of the thinness of the chest wall, breath sounds may seem much louder in children than in adults. Breath sounds in a child are almost all bronchovesicular or even bronchial, so that sound quality offers little help in diagnosis. Decreased breath sounds indicate decreased respiratory activity and are noted especially in children with bronchopneumonia, as well as with atelectasis, pleural effusion, pneumothorax and empyema. Increased breath sounds are sometimes heard with resolving pneumonia. The area over the mediastinum in the midline both anteriorly and posteriorly should be auscultated. Normally, no breath sounds will be heard over the sternum or vertebrae. Increased breath sounds will be heard in these areas in the presence of consolidation, foreign body, or tumor.

Inspiratory rales are usually heard as fine crackles. They may be heard scattered over the entire chest in infants and children with bronchiolitis, bronchopneumonia or atelectasis. Frequently, inspiratory rales are heard only at the very end of inspiration or only after deep inspiration. The crying child inspires deeply before each cry, so that auscultation may be quite informative during crying. The slightly older child may be instructed to blow against the examiner's hand; he will usually inspire deeply before blowing. The still older child can be instructed to breathe deeply through the mouth, especially if the examiner demonstrates this type of breathing.

Expiratory rales are usually heard as crackles during expiration. They are prominent in bronchiolitis, cystic fibrosis, asthma and foreign body aspiration. Fine rales are heard with pulmonary edema, which is rare in childhood.

The presence of fine rales may be clarified in children, as in adults, by having the patient cough at the end of expiration. Usually, the examiner should demonstrate exactly the procedure he expects the child to perform. Even small children can sometimes be induced to cough in this manner. Rales which disappear after coughing usually have no significance.

Pleural friction rub is a coarse grating sound heard through the stethoscope with each respiration as if it is close to the examiner's ear. It occurs occasionally with pneumonia, lung abscess, tuberculosis or empyema. A loud slap may be heard high on the chest in a child with a tracheal foreign body. A crunching sound near the heart and synchronous with the heart beat occurs with left pneumothorax, Hamman's sign.

Rhonchi due to crying or upper respiratory infection may be inspiratory or expiratory and are coarse sounds. They can best be distinguished from rales by tactile fremitus or by holding the bell stethoscope over the mouth and comparing the sounds from the mouth with those over the chest. If similar, the sounds are orig-

inating high in the respiratory tract near the larynx. Any
sound, especially if musical, which sounds the same over
different areas of the chest almost invariably arises from
the larynx or high in the trachea.

Wheezes usually sound more musical or sonorous
than rales or rhonchi. Wheezes are heard more commonly in expiration than in inspiration and usually indicate partial obstruction during the expiratory phase. Inspiratory wheezes usually are heard in children with high
obstruction such as laryngeal edema or foreign body and
expiratory wheezes are usually heard in children with low
obstruction such as asthma or bronchiolitis.

Vocal resonance can be obtained in children if they
are induced to count, speak, or tell their names repeatedly.
Increased resonance may indicate consolidation; and decreased resonance, obstruction to flow of air.

Peristalsis is frequently heard over the left lower
chest anteriorly due to the proximity of the bowel. However, peristalsis in the chest particularly on the left side
may be a cardinal sign of diaphragmatic hernia.

HEART

Certain basic information must be part of every examination of the heart. This includes rate, rhythm, size,
shape, quality of sounds, murmurs and thrills, femoral
pulses and blood pressure. In the routine examination of
the heart, it is advantageous to evaluate the patient in
several different positions if possible.

Inspection. - Observations made in the routine examination of the heart include note of the chest for precordial bulging, a sign of right-sided enlargement, and
the visible cardiac impulse, its localization and diffuse-
ness. Frequently, the cardiac impulse is noted in the
normal child or in a child who is hyperactive, thin or excited. It usually is not visible in many normal children.
If the impulse appears diffuse, it may be an indication of
cardiac enlargement or failure or it may be normal.
Noting the position of the impulse sometimes gives a rough
idea of the heart size, as it may correspond to the location
of the apex of the heart.

Other observations made as part of the routine examination of the heart include the appearance of respiratory distress, cyanosis, edema, clubbing of the fingers, capillary pulsations, prominence of veins, and abnormal pulsations of neck and epigastric veins. The presence or absence of femoral pulses and the obtaining of the blood pressure also help in determining the status of the heart.

Pulse. - The normal pulse rate in children varies from 70-170 at birth to 120-140 shortly after birth. Rates of 80-140 at one year, 80-130 at two years, 80-120 at three years and 70-115 after three years are within normal limits. Increased pulse rate may indicate excitement during examination, toxicity, fever from any cause, poor exercise tolerance due to congenital or acquired heart disease, digitalis intoxication, hyperthyroidism rarely, and other systemic diseases. Almost always, the pulse during sleep as well as day time is elevated in active rheumatic fever, any other active infection or thyrotoxicosis. In rheumatic fever, in contrast to other infections, the increased rate is usually out of proportion to the increase in temperature. The pulse rate is usually increased by 8-10 beats per minute for each degree of fever. In children with upper airway obstruction, pulse rates of 140-160 are common; in those with lower airway obstruction, rates may be 180-200 or higher.

Paroxysmal auricular tachycardia with rates as high as 200-300 per minute is sometimes noted in children with congenital heart disease or with toxic states. An idiopathic auricular tachycardia may be a cause of sudden death in infancy. Pulsus alternans, where one beat is strong and the next weak, is a sign of severe heart strain. A slow rate, bradycardia, most frequently means some degree of heart block, in infancy usually associated with a septal defect, digitalis poisoning, severe sepsis and, occasionally, hypothyroidism. In early teen-agers sinus bradycardia, especially with sinus arrhythmia, is common. Rare causes of slow pulse include carotid sinus hypersensitivity, hypercalcemia, increased intracranial pressure and, occasionally, acute myocarditis. The slow pulse rate sometimes seen in children with hypertension in acute nephritis may be related to an associated increased intracranial pressure.

Water-hammer or Corrigan pulse is felt as an especially forceful beat due to a very wide pulse pressure. It is noted best either over the radial or femoral arteries. Capillary pulsations, or Quinke pulse, noted most easily after pressing lightly on the tip of the nail, also are due to increased pulse pressure. A method sometimes used for eliciting capillary pulsations is the rubbing of the skin of the forehead vigorously for a minute until generalized erythema appears. Observation reveals intermittent reddening and blanching in children with increased capillary pressures. Both of these pulse types are found especially in older children with patent ductus arteriosus, aortic regurgitation or peripheral arteriovenous fistula.

Thready pulse is a rapid, weak pulse which seems to appear and disappear. It is usually a sign of circulatory failure, shock or heart failure. A dicrotic pulse is a pulse which feels as if it has a notch in it. The normal pulse has this notch but it cannot usually be palpated. It may be found in children with typhoid fever or other sepsis. Pulsus paradoxus is a marked change in pulse amplitude with respiration. It may be felt normally in children with well-developed thoracic respiration or may be a sign of the rarely occurring cardiac tamponade due to pericardial effusion or constrictive pericarditis.

Almost all children, especially young adolescents, normally have sinus arrhythmia. Occasional runs of premature beats or of extrasystoles are not uncommon in childhood and may have no clinical significance. Regular rhythm in childhood is not rare but if present, may indicate active rheumatic fever or other active carditis. One rarely sees auricular fibrillation in childhood because the chief cause of this, rheumatic heart disease, develops in older children or adults following the childhood rheumatic fever.

Measurement of the size of the heart gives one the best idea of the presence of heart disease. Measurement of heart size by physical examination alone may be difficult in childhood, but estimation of size can be made with careful inspection, palpation and percussion.

Palpation. - Palpation is useful in detecting the apex

impulse (point of maximum impulse, PMI) of the heart.
While the PMI is an important physical sign which usually
indicates the location of the apex of the heart, a more reliable guide to the position of the apex is the apex beat.
This is the position farthest toward the axilla and toward
the lower rib margin which can be easily palpated. This
is normally at the fifth interspace in the midclavicular line
after the age of seven years. Before this age, the apex
impulse is normally felt in the fourth interspace just to the
left of the midclavicular line. The apex is usually at a
lower interspace and more lateral in children with cardiac
enlargement; however, pericardial effusion or various
lung, spine and chest wall diseases may also displace
the apex.

The apex impulse may be difficult to feel in children
less than two years of age, or in children with pericardial
effusion, heart failure or emphysema. A forceful apex
beat is felt in children after exercise, in children with
thin chest walls, with excitement, impending heart failure, fever or hyperthyroidism.

Occasionally, right ventricular hypertrophy can be
distinguished from left ventricular hypertrophy by palpation. With left ventricle hypertrophy, the apex impulse
feels diffuse and heaving; with right hypertrophy, usually
the impulse is felt as a sharp tap. Usually the first (systolic) sound, occasionally the second (diastolic) sound and
in a failing heart a third sound (gallop rhythm) may be
palpated.

Occasionally, the child will complain of tenderness
when the heart area is palpated. This does not mean that
heart disease is present or absent.

Vibratory thrills and pericardial friction rubs may
also be palpated. They are felt as fine or coarse vibrations, either continuously or during some part of the cardiac cycle. Position of cardiac thrills and their timing in
the cardiac cycle should be recorded. Timing can be obtained by simultaneously feeling either the apex impulse or
the carotid pulse. Thrills at the apex are more easily felt
with the child on the left side; and basal thrills with the
child sitting up.

Systolic thrills at the base of the heart are usually due to septal defects, aortic stenosis or, occasionally, pulmonary stenosis. Continuous thrill at the base of the heart may be due to patent ductus arteriosus. A diastolic thrill at the apex is usually due to mitral stenosis.

Percussion. - Percussion of the heart, as percussion of the lungs, may be performed by either the direct or the indirect method. Scratch-percussion is sometimes used to determine cardiac borders. With the stethoscope over the heart, longitudinal parallel scratches are made with the finger beginning in the axillary line, and moving toward the heart at about one-quarter inch intervals. As soon as the scratches are being made over the heart, a change in intensity of the scratch sound will be detected through the stethoscope (Fig. 17).

A combined method of palpation and auscultation may be found even more satisfactory for estimating heart size and shape. The stethoscope is placed firmly on the chest just to the right of the sternum. The chest wall is tapped lightly with the index finger, beginning in the axillary line and coming medially. As soon as the finger is tapping over the heart, an immediate intensification of sound will be heard.

Fig. 17. Scratch percussion. The stethoscope is near the sternum; parallel scratches are made down the left side of the chest.

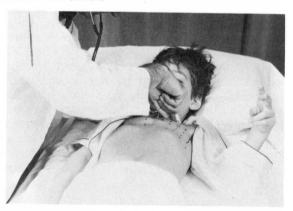

The heart is usually percussed easily as a triangular area with one side of the triangle extending along the right sternal border from the second to the fifth rib, one side being a line from the right sternal to the midclavicular line along the fifth rib, and the hypotenuse being the line from the right sternal border at the second rib to the midclavicular line at the fifth rib. Normally, the heart of the infant is usually more horizontal, and the apex of the left border dullness (LBD) is to the left of the nipple line.

The area of heart dullness may be altered in a child with a normal or abnormal heart size. The heart may be percussed at a lower interspace or more lateral-ward with right or left ventricular hypertrophy. Percussion dullness to the right of the sternum in the third or fourth interspace usually indicates right-sided heart enlargement. In children with emphysema or space-taking lesions in the chest, the heart will be pushed away from the lesion; while in children with atelectasis, the heart will be pulled toward the side of the lesion. The heart is percussed on the right side of the chest in children with dextrocardia. The heart normally moves a little as the patient is turned from side to side. If motion does not occur when the patient is turned, pulmonary masses or adhesions may be present. This physical finding is rare in childhood. The heart may be percussed far to the left in the second and third interspace when the child is recumbent, and in the normal position when he sits. This may indicate the presence of pericardial effusion.

Small hearts, characteristic of patients with Addison's disease or constrictive pericarditis, are rarely seen in childhood. An enlarged heart is characteristic of almost all types of heart disease: congenital heart disease with heart strain, anemia, myocarditis or rheumatic fever. Less common causes of enlarged heart include endocardial fibro-elastosis; pericardial effusion, patent ductus arteriosus, hypertension in nephritis, tumors, glycogen storage disease or peripheral arteriovenous shunt. Patent ductus arteriosus may be present with a normal-sized heart.

It is important to try to determine whether the right or left side of the heart is enlarged. This is difficult by physical examination alone. Right-sided enlargement pro-

duces precordial bulging and may be accompanied by characteristic palpatory findings. It is characteristic of such
conditions as inter-atrial septal defect or pulmonic stenosis or, in older children, mitral stenosis. Right-sided
strain in general is more common with congenital heart
lesions, though left-sided failure is seen with coarctation
of the aorta, tricuspid atresia, endocardial fibro-elastosis,
glycogen storage disease, aberrant origin of the coronary
arteries or aberrant pulmonary veins.

Auscultation. - Auscultation is performed in a manner
similar to auscultation of the lungs. The entire precordium
is auscultated with special reference to the valve areas as
in adults: the areas listed (Fig. 18) are the listening posts
of the valve areas, and not the true or anatomical valve
areas. These areas regularly include the mitral valve at
the apex, the pulmonary valve at the second interspace to
the left of the sternum, the aortic valve at the second interspace to the right of the sternum (and at the third left interspace for diastolic murmurs), and the tricuspid valve in
the fourth interspace over the sternum. In addition to these
areas, it is just as important to auscultate in children just
to the right of the apex and several cm. to the left of the
sternum in the third interspace (frequent sites of functional
murmurs), along the sternal border (murmurs of septal

Fig. 18.   Listening areas of the heart.

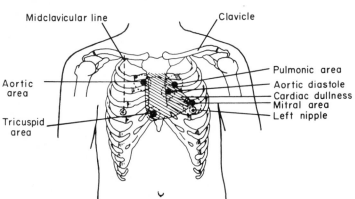

defects), second and third interspaces several cm. to the left of the sternum (murmurs of patent ductus arteriosus and coarctation of the aorta), above the clavicles (venous hums and transmitted murmurs), and in the axillae, along the left midaxillary line, and below the scapulae (transmitted murmurs). Auscultation usually gives a better count of the cardiac rate than palpation at the wrist in children.

The quality of the sounds is important. The first sound is due to mitral and tricuspid (atrioventricular) valve closure and is best heard over these valve areas. When the first sound is split, the first component is due to mitral closure. The second sound is due to aortic and pulmonic valve closure, the aortic valve closing slightly before the pulmonic. Splitting of the second sound is heard best in the pulmonic area and is common in normal children. The split widens on inspiration. Deep inspiration delays pulmonic valve closure and increases the splitting of the second sound. The first sound is best heard with the bell and the second with the diaphragm. In the newborn they may normally be distant and difficult to obtain. The sounds should be sharp and clear. Distant sounds may indicate pericardial fluid, atelectasis or other pulmonary disease. Sounds of poor quality are those which do not sound clear but are slurred or "mushy." These sounds almost always are characteristic of severe heart disease or myocarditis, usually with heart failure. In the newborn, both sounds are of about equal intensity. Later the apical first sound is louder than the second and the pulmonic second sound is louder than the first in childhood.

A loud snapping apical first sound is heard with mitral stenosis. A decreased apical first sound is heard in early myocarditis. Decreased or absent pulmonary second sound usually occurs with pulmonic stenosis. The pulmonic second sound is normally louder than the aortic second sound during childhood. The pulmonic second sound often is heard better in the third than in the second left interspace in children. The aortic second sound is usually diminished in intensity with aortic stenosis and acute myocarditis. With aortic insufficiency, the aortic second sound is often increased, but it may be decreased or absent. The aortic second sound is increased in children with hypertension from any cause. The tricuspid first sound may be obliterated with tricuspid regurgitation, a rare congenital anomaly.

Either the first or second sound may be split in any valvular area without causing concern, and a third heart sound is present in about one-third of all children. Four criteria are useful in distinguishing split sounds from a third heart sound: intensity and quality, position heard, and distance between sounds. Split second sounds are of equal quality and intensity, are heard most frequently at the base of the heart, and occur with a very short interval between the sounds. The third sound is best heard at the apex, with a longer interval between the second and third sounds, and usually with differing intensities and qualities. Split second sounds at the base of the heart are common in children with conditions causing left to right shunts. Splitting at the base is absent in children with pulmonic stenosis. The wide splitting characteristically heard in children with atrial septal defects remains constant during inspiration and expiration.

It is occasionally difficult to distinguish the third heart sound from a gallop rhythm which indicates a failing heart. Occasionally, the three beats of the gallop can be felt on palpation; the third heart sound can never be felt as an impulse. Usually differentiation between third sound and gallop rhythm is based on the presence of other evidence of heart disease, when gallop rhythm would be more likely than a third heart sound. Tic-tac rhythm, embryocardia, exists if both sounds are almost alike in quality and intensity and are equidistant from each other. While normal in the younger child, this rhythm in the older child may indicate a failing heart.

Pericardial friction rub is a grating to-and-fro sound heard through the stethoscope as if it is close to the examiner's ear and is increased by pressure of the stethoscope on the chest or by the patient leaning forward. Intensity of the rub varies with the phase of the cardiac cycle. Rub usually indicates pericarditis, particularly

that due to tuberculosis or acute rheumatic fever, and
sometimes may be detected on palpation as a vibratory
thrill. Pleuropericardial rubs are more common than
pericardial rubs. They are heard best in the manner described, but they are noted to vary with the phase of respiration rather than with cardiac activity. They may be
confused with pericardial rubs, usually have no pathological
significance, may be caused by the proximity of the heart
and lungs, but may indicate pleuropericardial adhesions.

Venous hum is a continuous low-pitched sound originating in the internal jugular vein, heard sometimes over
the clavicles. It usually radiates downward, has no pathological significance, but must be distinguished from a
murmur. The hum is usually louder when the patient is
sitting, disappears in recumbency, and may be abolished
by pressure on the internal jugular vein. Venous hums
over the abdomen, especially near the umbilicus, are
sometimes heard in children with cirrhosis of the liver or
portal obstruction.

Perhaps the most difficult diagnostic feature in the
physical examination of a child is the determination of the
significance of murmurs. Many children have murmurs
without heart disease, and occasionally newborn infants
or others have severe heart disease with no murmurs.
Systolic murmurs are those coming at or after the first
and before the second sound; diastolic murmurs come at
or after the second and before the first sound. Murmurs
heard in systole are early systolic, late systolic, or
throughout systole (holosystolic). Diastolic murmurs
may be early (protodiastolic), mid-diastolic, or late in
diastole (presystolic).

The quality of the murmurs is noted as soft, harsh,
blowing, whistling, etc. The intensity of the murmurs
should be graded. According to one system of grading,
a grade I murmur is the softest possible murmur heard.
It is not heard in all positions, especially not when the
patient sits up or after he exercises. A grade II murmur
is the weakest murmur heard in all positions or after
exercise. A grade III murmur is a loud murmur but not
accompanied by a thrill. A grade IV murmur is a loud

murmur with a thrill. A grade V murmur is a murmur heard with the stethoscope barely on the chest. A grade VI murmur can be heard with the stethoscope not touching the chest!

The intensity of murmurs alone does not indicate whether the murmur is significant of heart disease, though murmurs of grade III or louder usually indicate heart disease. Following the intensity of a murmur over a period of hours, days or weeks is helpful in determining the course of the heart disease. This is especially true in rheumatic fever and bacterial endocarditis where the quality of the murmurs may change rapidly.

Murmurs may "rumble" for a short distance around the site of maximum intensity of the murmur, but "radiate" or are said to be transmitted if they are heard with good intensity some distance away from the site of maximum intensity. Innocent murmurs usually do not radiate, and they may change in character with change in position or phase of respiration. Innocent murmurs may appear or disappear during fever, exercise, excitement or anemia. They vary with respiration. A diastolic murmur or a murmur which is transmitted or radiates indicates heart disease unless proved otherwise. Cardiopulmonary murmurs are soft, high-pitched sounds caused by the apposition of the heart and lungs, occur always in the same phase of respiration, can be obliterated by changing position, usually have no pathological significance, but may indicate the presence of pleural adhesions.

Ordinarily, short blowing early or mid-systolic murmurs of low pitch heard best in the pulmonary area or musical buzzing vibratory murmurs over the precordium are innocent. If these murmurs radiate they usually radiate downward, whereas if murmurs of mitral insufficiency radiate they usually radiate laterally. Also, the murmur of mitral insufficiency is continual and is at or lateral to the apex, whereas the innocent murmur which is short is usually medial to the apex in the general area where the murmurs of septal defects are heard. A holo-systolic crescendo-decrescendo loud harsh murmur over the pulmonic area is characteristic of pulmonic stenosis and is heard also with atrial septal defects or anomalous pulmonary venous return. This type of "diamond-shaped" murmur, which reaches its peak loudness in the middle third of systole is termed "ejection-type," may be associated with ejection clicks and indicates pulmonary, aortic or infundibular stenosis. Holo-systolic murmurs are caused by blood flow from a chamber with higher to a chamber with lower pressure, and are regurgitant. They are common with mitral or tricuspid valve incompetence and septal defects. Detection of this murmur very early in systole distinguishes it from innocent murmur.

Those diastolic murmurs which start loud and then diminish in intensity are decrescendo, e. g. , the murmur of aortic or pulmonic insufficiency. At the base of the heart those starting softly and increasing in intensity are crescendo murmurs, e. g. , those murmurs of mitral or tricuspid stenosis due either to valvular disease or to increased flow secondary to a left-to-right shunt. Presystolic murmurs are usually associated with active atrial contraction plus stenosis of the mitral or tricuspid valve.

The murmurs of septal defects and pulmonic stenosis may be heard alone as isolated congenital anomalies or in combination, as in the tetralogy of Fallot.

A continuous murmur in the second or third interspace to the left of the sternum and widely transmitted is characteristic of patent ductus arteriosus. A hum or high-pitched murmur anywhere along the course of the aorta may be due to coarctation of the aorta or, rarely, a thrombosis of the aorta. A continuous murmur in the right or left parasternal areas may indicate a coronary or other arteriovenous fistula.

Rheumatic carditis is a type of acquired heart disease. A harsh systolic high-pitched or soft blow, sometimes obliterating the first sound and lasting through systole up to the second sound, or beginning in late systole with crescendo to the second sound, at or just to the right of the apex, may be the first sign of carditis and is usually due to mitral insufficiency. This murmur is usually transmitted to the axilla or back. Later, an early or mid-diastolic crescendo blow in the same area with a loud mitral first sound may indicate relative mitral stenosis --

relative because of the disproportion of the size of the
valve and the ventricle. These murmurs disappear when
the carditis disappears. The murmur of true mitral
stenosis is similar except that, in addition, early in diastole a snap is heard due to mitral valve opening. A
later snap in diastole occurs with pericarditis and must
be distinguished from the third heart sound. Late signs
are the blowing diastolic decrescendo murmur of aortic
insufficiency, heard best with the diaphragm stethoscope
just to the left of the sternum in the third interspace.
This murmur may radiate down the left sternal border.
A systolic high-pitched murmur in the second interspace
to the right of the sternum, transmitted to the neck with
a decreased aortic second sound and often a thrill, is
usually due to aortic stenosis. A systolic high-pitched
murmur in the third left interspace, with a decreased
pulmonic second sound, is usually due to pulmonic stenosis. Tricuspid murmurs are rare; tricuspid murmurs
are similar in character to mitral murmurs; a systolic
murmur indicates tricuspid insufficiency and a diastolic
murmur, tricuspid stenosis.

The murmurs heard in the tricuspid area and the
murmur of pulmonic stenosis are more often due to congenital than to acquired anomalies during childhood. The
murmur of aortic stenosis is frequently due to a congenital lesion, and the murmur of aortic insufficiency is
rarely heard during childhood, as aortic insufficiency
develops late in the course of rheumatic carditis.

In general, the type of heart disease is not diagnosed
by examination alone. One first makes a tentative diagnosis by history and repeated observation and tries to confirm or eliminate this diagnosis by the examination and
suitable laboratory studies.

For example, a child under five years of age rarely
has rheumatic fever, and even if over five years of age he
should have other characteristic signs of rheumatic fever
such as joint pains, subcutaneous nodules, chorea or erythema nodosum. Even in an older child without fever or
increased pulse rate this diagnosis is not very likely,
though possible. If a child has fever, increased pulse
rate, and murmurs, one also has to consider the diagno-

sis of fever with innocent murmurs or myocarditis secondary to infection elsewhere as in nephritis, diphtheria or tonsillitis.

Next, one considers in a child under five years whether the heart disease is cyanotic or acyanotic.

Severe cyanosis at birth which has been determined, as described in the chapter on the Newborn, to be due to heart disease, usually indicates one of the most severe congenital heart lesions such as transposition of the great vessels, truncus arteriosus or tricuspid atresia. Cyanosis developing later in the first year of life is due to an increasing shunt from the right heart to the left such as occurs in tetralogy of Fallot where the increasing pulmonic stenosis causes increasing right ventricular pressure. Cyanosis developing at four or five years of age may indicate Eisenmenger's complex or pulmonic stenosis with septal defect. If cyanosis is not present unless the child exercises or cries, an atrial septal defect without pulmonic stenosis is suggested, as the right-sided pressure is not increased until the intrapulmonary pressure is increased by crying.

The important non-cyanotic heart diseases of infancy are toxic myocarditis from any cause, endocardial fibroelastosis, tumors of the heart and, most commonly, patent ductus arteriosus and coarctation of the aorta. Patent ductus arteriosus has a characteristic murmur and high pulse pressure, and coarctation of the aorta has a normal or high pressure in the arms, very low pressure in the legs, and absent or weak femoral pulses. Other non-cyanotic heart lesions, such as right aortic arch, dextroposition of the heart and aortic vascular ring, are diagnosed by examination and by history suggesting obstruction of the trachea or esophagus by an extrinsic mass.

It is important to realize also that the <u>signs of heart failure</u> in young children are not similar to those in adults. Early, one sees only a rapid respiratory rate in the supine position, followed by slight dyspnea. The liver becomes enlarged early and there may be venous engorgement and orthopnea; pulsus alternans and gallop rhythm, if present, are almost pathognomonic of heart failure. Only late does one find signs of pulmonary or peripheral edema.

CHAPTER VI

The Abdomen

Frequently the abdomen is examined first. This requires few instruments which may frighten the child. Naturally, it is impossible to do a thorough examination if the child is afraid or crying, or if the abdominal wall is taut. Sometimes, it is necessary to examine parts of the abdomen while the child is quiet and come back to the abdomen again as the child quiets again. Warm the hands before examining the abdomen. If the child is ticklish, have him place his hand over your palpating hand.

Inspection. - First, the abdomen is inspected. The shape is noted. Ordinarily, the abdominal musculature is thinner than that of the adult and the child has a lordotic stance, giving the appearance of a "pot-belly." This appearance can generally be regarded as normal until the child reaches puberty.

Real distention of the abdomen is caused usually by air or fluid in the bowel or peritoneal cavity, but may also be caused by atonic abdominal musculature, paralysis of the abdominal musculature, feces in the bowel, abnormal enlargement of organs, intestinal duplication, or tumors. Children with pancreatic fibrosis, hypokalemia, rickets, hypothyroidism, bowel obstruction, constipation, ileus, or ascites are especially prone to show abdominal distention. Transillumination of the abdomen with a strong light beam should be performed to differentiate cystic from solid masses in a child with an enlarged abdomen. Transillumination helps detect cystic tumors, bladder distention, and multicystic or hydronephrotic kidneys, as well as ascites.

Respiration is largely abdominal in children up to six or seven years of age and, even after this age, the abdominal wall usually moves with respiration when the child is in the supine position. If the abdominal wall fails to move with respiration, peritonitis, appendicitis, other acute surgical emergencies of the abdomen, paralytic ileus, diaphragmatic paralysis, a large amount of ascitic fluid or a large amount of abdominal air may be present. If respiration is entirely abdominal in the young child, or largely abdominal in the older child, emphysema, pneumonia or other pulmonary disorder should be suspected.

The abdomen is normally flat when the child is in the supine position. Occasionally, however, the abdomen will appear depressed or scaphoid. In the newborn, this may signify a large diaphragmatic hernia with most of the abdominal contents in the chest. In older children, scaphoid abdomen occurs with marked dehydration or high intestinal obstruction. With pneumothorax, the chest is large and the abdomen, though normal, may appear to be scaphoid.

The umbilicus is observed. Normally, it is closed and puckered but hernia may be present as observed by protrusion of some abdominal contents. Umbilical hernias are common in all infants up to the age of two years, and in Negro children up to the age of seven years. Hernias are especially common in children with hypothyroidism, mongolism, the chondrodystrophies, or with large chronically distended abdomens. Granulomas, ulcers, and drainage of the umbilicus occur in the newborn and are discussed later. Umbilical hernias and diastasis of the recti can frequently be observed, if present, when the child cries or coughs.

Diastasis of the rectus muscles may be noted as a protrusion in the midline, usually from the xiphoid to the umbilicus, but occasionally down to the symphysis pubis. Ordinarily, the protrusion is one-half to two inches wide; it is usually a normal variant but may be due to a congenital weakness of the musculature or to chronically distended abdomen.

Paradoxical motion of the umbilicus is noted with unilateral or asymmetrical paralysis of the abdominal wall musculature or of one part of the diaphragm.

The veins are noted. In small infants with good subcutaneous tissue, veins are rarely visible. Visible but not
distended veins are usually noted until puberty in normal
children and are especially noticeable in malnourished
children. Distended veins are seen with heart failure,
peritonitis or venous obstruction. Direction of flow of
blood in dilated veins should be noted. Blood flow from
the veins below the umbilicus, normally downward, is
usually reversed in children with obstruction of the inferior vena cava or with portal hypertension. Diffuse
epigastric pulsations may be noted normally, or may indicate right ventricular hypertrophy with transmission of
the pulsations through the diaphragm.

Next one looks for peristalsis. Peristalsis is most
easily seen if the examiner's eye is about at the level of
the abdomen and a light is directed across the abdomen.
Moving shadows will be noted in the presence of excessive peristalsis. Visible peristalsis is always a sign of
obstruction until ruled otherwise. It may be seen normally in thin small infants, especially premature ones.
In infants up to two months of age visible peristalsis may
indicate pyloric stenosis or pylorospasm, but one cannot
distinguish the type of obstruction by the nature of the
visible peristalsis. Gastric waves, which pass from left
to right, usually indicate pyloric stenosis.

Auscultation. Next, one auscultates the abdomen
and listens for peristalsis. It is better to auscultate the
abdomen before proceeding with the examination not only
because one frequently forgets to listen if he postpones
this part of the examination, but also because manipulation done later may so alter peristaltic sounds that a true
appraisal becomes impossible.

Peristaltic sounds are normally heard as metallic
short tinkling. A sound may be heard normally every ten
to thirty seconds. The examiner must place the stethoscope firmly over the abdomen and listen carefully, as the
sounds normally may be of low intensity. Sounds may be
increased in frequency and intensity simply by stroking
the abdomen with a finger nail. They are high pitched
and frequent in early peritonitis, diarrhea from any cause,

intestinal obstruction, or gastroenteritis. Peristaltic
sounds are absent in paralytic ileus and may be decreased
to absent in children with early peritonitis. Listening to
the abdomen and hearing the typical sounds of peritonitis
may be the only way of detecting pneumococcal peritonitis
in nephrosis or in other conditions where there is free
fluid in the abdomen. Free fluid may give one the impression of a non-tense abdomen even though peritonitis is
present. Rarely, a venous hum may be heard during
auscultation, as a sign of portal obstruction. A murmur
may be heard over the abdomen in children with coarctation of the aorta. The area over the kidneys should be
auscultated posteriorly with the bell stethoscope in children with hypertension. A murmur in this area may suggest constriction of one of the renal arteries.

Percussion. - After auscultating the abdomen, one
percusses by the indirect method previously described.
A tympanitic sound in a distended abdomen signifies that
gas is present in the abdomen. Tympanites, or an unusually tympanitic sound, is common with low intestinal
obstruction, air-swallowing, or paralytic ileus.

A distended abdomen with little tympany suggests
fluid or solid masses. When one suspects fluid, he should
test also for fluid wave and shifting dullness. Fluid wave
is obtained with difficulty in children. It may be elicited
in the following manner. The edge of an aide's hand is
placed firmly along the midline of the abdomen. One of
the examiner's hands is placed on one side of the patient's
abdomen. The other hand of the examiner strikes sharply
the opposite side of the patient's abdomen, and a wave is
felt against the first hand as if it arises from deep in the
abdomen. Shifting dullness is most easily obtained by
percussing and delineating the area of dullness with the
patient in one position. Then, the position of the patient
is changed, and dullness again elicited. Slight shifting
dullness is normal or may be found with tumors, but considerable shift is usually obtained in patients with free
abdominal fluid. Fluid in the abdomen, ascites, is found
in children with chronic liver disease (e.g., cirrhosis),
chronic kidney disease (e.g., nephrosis), tuberculous

peritonitis and, rarely, with heart failure or with rupture or other leak of the abdominal lymphatics, chylous ascites.

Solid masses, described later, will also be percussed. Frequently a dull percussion note indicates a mass which cannot be felt. One should also note that there is always dullness to percussion in the area of the liver, except if free air is present in the abdominal cavity.

Palpation. - There are several satisfactory methods of palpating the abdomen, though all methods should consider the comfort of patient and physician.

The patient should be distracted during abdominal palpation by unrelated conversation or other means. The abdomen may be palpated with the child asleep. This is especially helpful if an acute abdomen is suspected. If the patient will cooperate, he can be asked to take deep breaths and to flex his knees during this part of the examination. Palpation is best performed if it can be done in inspiration and deep expiration. One hand is placed flat on the back of the patient, and the other on the anterior surface of the abdomen. First, one palpates gently and superficially, using the upper hand for most of the palpatory sensation. One begins in the left lower quadrant and then proceeds to the left upper, right upper and right lower quadrants; but if a localized site of pain or tenderness is found, this area should be palpated after the other parts of the abdomen have been palpated.

One notes first whether the abdomen is soft or hard. With a tense abdomen, there is a feeling of marked rigidity or resistance to pressure. A hard tense abdomen immediately directs the examiner to consider a surgical condition, any condition which may produce tenderness or, rarely, such states as tetanus or hypoparathyroidism. In a crying child, one can distinguish between a soft and hard abdomen, by feeling immediately on inspiration, when the child may relax for an instant. If the child is tense and does not relax, and a question of abdominal pathology exists, the child of any age can be placed in a warm tub. This may relax the abdomen enough to feel masses or to localize tenderness or rigidity.

Tenderness is noted and the point of maximal tender-

ness must be determined. Frequently a patient will say an
area is tender and the examiner will doubt the accuracy of
the statement. In such a case it is best to touch a completely neutral area such as the thigh and ask the patient if
that area is tender. One should not ask the patient "Does
this hurt?" unless he is old enough to be completely reliable. Rather, one can easily determine the site of tenderness by watching the patient's face, noting wincing, cry,
and change of pitch of cry as the really tender area is
touched. When asked where the abdomen hurts, a young
child almost always points to the umbilicus. Pointing to
any other part may be significant. Tenderness can be further localized by noting pain on rebound. The examiner
places one hand deep in the abdomen, away from the suspected area of tenderness and quickly removes his hand.
The child may again complain of pain in the area originally
under suspicion.

In general, even localized tenderness is not well cor-
related with underlying pathology. Tenderness in the lower
quadrants may be due to such states as gastroenteritis,
feces, obstruction, tumor or, rarely, a Meckel's diverticulum with ulceration, torsion of the ovary, or torsion of
the testis. Lower abdominal tenderness after a menstrual
period may be due to pelvic infection. Tenderness in the
right lower quadrant may be due to appendicitis or abscess;
in the right upper quadrant, acutely enlarged liver, hepatitis or intussusception; in the left upper quadrant, acute
splenic enlargement, intussusception or splenic rupture.
Midline tenderness in the upper abdomen may be due to
gastroenteritis, coughing, vomiting, gastric or duodenal
ulcer; in the midline of the lower abdomen marked superficial tenderness may be diagnostic of cystitis, but deep
tenderness may be due to the palpation of the normal
aorta. Intra-abdominal tenderness can be distinguished
from muscle tenderness by asking the child to raise his
head and then palpating. Intra-abdominal tenderness is
lessened, while superficial tenderness is increased, by
this maneuver.

Poorly localized areas of abdominal tenderness may
be due to pneumonia, upper respiratory infection, mesen-

teric adenitis, peritonitis, rheumatic fever, measles, crisis of sickle-cell anemia, leukemia, allergy, acidosis, emotional crisis, other infections or ruptured viscus.

If the abdominal wall is not tense, one feels for the superficial masses. The enlarged spleen is usually felt as a superficial mass in the left upper quadrant. It may feel like a tongue hanging from the left costal margin with a sharp straight border and a notch on the anterior margin. Splenic enlargement is found in children with such diseases as septicemia, other infections, blood dyscrasias including sickle-cell anemia, thalassemia major, hemolytic jaundice, infectious mononucleosis and leukemia, the reticuloendothelioses, or the connective tissue diseases. A very large spleen with less enlarged liver also is seen with portal vein obstruction and in neonatal hepatitis. It may be normally palpable 1-2 cm. below the left costal margin in the first few weeks of life due to extra-medullary hematopoiesis, and also in normal infants and young children. Its size should be noted; and also whether or not it is tender. Floating ribs are sometimes confused with the spleen on palpation. Usually differentiation can be made by simultaneous palpation bilaterally or by percussion.

The liver is generally palpable as a superficial mass 1-2 cm. below the right costal margin, with a sharp border during the first year. Size, consistency, tenderness and pulsation are noted. It may remain palpable during childhood without pathological significance. If more than 2 cm. below the costal margin, it may indicate such states as passive congestion, hepatitis, tumor or metastases, blood dyscrasias, septicemia or other infections, the reticuloendothelial or metabolic diseases or pulmonary emphysema. Rapidly enlarging liver is an early sign of right heart failure. The liver edge is usually not as sharp in failure as it is in pulmonary emphysema without failure. Rapidly decreasing liver size may be diagnostic of acute liver necrosis. A thrill felt over an enlarged liver is found with hydatid echinococcal cysts in the liver; a gurgling sound may be heard in the same area. Pulsation of the liver is usually due to transmission of the impulse from the aorta, but quite rarely it may be due to tricuspid regurgitation or stenosis, or to constrictive pericarditis.

Other masses such as neuroblastoma, Wilms's tumor, duplication of the intestinal tract and urinary bladder, circumscribed collections of blood, collection of fluid in the uterus due to an imperforate hymen, hydrometrocolpos, or an enlarged uterus due to pregnancy may be palpated superficially. The spleen can be pushed medially, laterally, and upward if necessary to distinguish it from an enlarged left lobe of the liver. It may be felt superficial to the colon, distinguishing it from a retroperitoneal mass. Wilms's tumor may be distinguished from a neuroblastoma as Wilms's ordinarily does not cross the midline. Ovarian tumors palpated in pre-adolescent girls may be malignant; after the menarche they are more likely to be functional.

After superficial palpation, one proceeds in the same manner around the quadrants of the abdomen, but palpates more deeply, using the posterior hand to push masses forward. The anterior hand pushes down so that the skin of the anterior abdomen is actually indented one to two inches. In children with ascites, it may be difficult to feel any masses directly. However, percussion may indicate a few areas of increased dullness, and palpation by ballottement should delineate a few of the larger masses. In ballotting (Fig. 19) one places one hand lightly above the area to be ballotted, and one hand firmly below the area to be ballotted. With the ballotting hand, one quickly flicks the area. If a ballottable mass is present, a rebound sensation will be felt in the ballotting hand, as if a ball has been thrown forward and comes back.

In addition to delineating the masses already noted, one looks for certain special masses. For example, the tumor of pyloric stenosis is best felt on deep palpation after the infant vomits. This mass is usually located at the end of the stomach anywhere along the edge of the liver from the costal margin in the midline to the underside of the right lobe of the liver. The sausage-shaped tender mass of intussusception can usually be palpated in the right lower quadrant. Other masses such as those due to

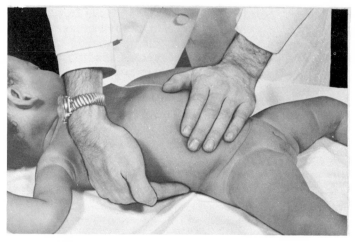

Fig. 19.   Ballotting for right kidney.

urinary tract anomalies such as malposition, hydro-ureter, or hydronephrosis, and the filled bladder may be palpated. Bladder enlargement may be due to many types of urinary tract obstruction, to voluntary control or embarrassment of the patient, or to low spinal cord lesions.

By placing the index finger in the costovertebral angle and pushing up gently but sharply as in ballottement, one can usually palpate about one or two cm. of the right kidney and frequently the tip of the left kidney. The reverse procedure even more frequently allows one to feel the normal as well as the enlarged kidney. The abdomen of the child in the supine position is gently elevated with one hand, and all the fingers of the other hand are placed flat over the back of the elevated side so that the index finger lies in the costovertebral angle. The hand which is holding the abdomen is released and as the side of the abdomen falls toward the mattress, the kidney will hit the hand on the back. Enlarged kidneys usually indicate infection, congenital anomaly, tumor of the kidney or renal vein thrombosis.

It should be remembered that a few children will have malrotation of the organs, as in situs inversus or

congenital malrotation. In children who have had oper-
ations for repair of omphalocele, and sometimes for diaphragmatic hernia, the organs are so displaced that it
may be impossible to recognize even normal organs.

Every mass in the abdomen must be explained adequately before a patient can be considered free of disease. Occasionally, however, one mistakes feces in a
child who is not even constipated, or the abdominal aorta,
for an abnormal mass.

One palpates also for a diastasis between the rectus
muscles. The umbilical hernia previously noted should
be palpated. One notes the presence of bowel in the hernia
by palpating a gas-filled loop and by obtaining the feeling
of silk rubbing against silk on replacing the viscus. If the
hernia cannot be easily reduced, this is also noted. Finally
one should make careful note of the size of the hernia.

Abdominal reflexes are tested. These are obtained
by scratching the skin of the abdomen with four scratches
to make a diamond, the points of the diamond being the
midline shortly below the xiphoid and above the symphysis,
and both sides of the abdomen at the level of the umbilicus.
The umbilicus normally moves at each scratch. This reflex is absent in normal children under one year of age and
in children with early poliomyelitis or with multiple sclerosis or other central or pyramidal disorder.

One next palpates the inguinal and femoral regions
for hernias, lymph nodes and femoral pulses (Fig. 20).
Femoral pulses are best felt by placing the tips of two or
three fingers along the inguinal ligament about midway
between the iliac crest and symphysis pubis. With gentle
pressure, definite pulsation should be felt by one of the
fingers. Alternatively, direct pressure on the two or
three fingers by the fingers of the free hand may make
it easier to feel the pulse. Absent femoral pulse indicates coarctation of the aorta. Auscultation over the
femoral artery may reveal a booming sound or "pistol
shot" characteristic of aortic insufficiency or other causes
of increased pulse pressure. A double sound (Traube's
double tone) is indicative of the same. A systolic and
diastolic murmur may also be heard in these conditions

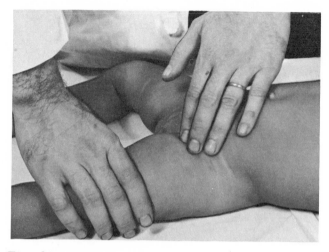

Fig. 20.   Palpating femoral area for femoral pulse.

(Duroziez's sign).   Hernias are palpated in a special
manner described below.

One of the favorite sites of determining dehydration
in a child is over the abdomen.   One should pull up about
two or three inches of the skin and subcutaneous tissue,
and quickly release it.   If the creases formed by pulling
the skin do not disappear immediately, dehydration is
present.

Occasionally, the wall of the abdomen feels putty-
like in consistency.   This may be normal, but it occurs
especially in children who are chronically malnourished
or dehydrated, or in children with such diseases as peritonitis, tuberculous peritonitis, the reticuloendothelioses,
myxedema or hyperelectrolytemia.

GENITALIA

One learns much about genitalia simply by looking.
Urethral discharges are always pathological in childhood
and may indicate infection anywhere in the urinary tract.
A flaming red area at the end of the urethra may be due

to prolapse of the urethral mucosa. A cyst may be present at the urethral meatus in either sex.

A bloody <u>vaginal discharge</u> is normal, but not common, up to the fourth week of life. Vaginal bleeding in children less than eight years old is usually due either to foreign bodies, injury, or to constitutional isosexual precocity of unknown cause; ovarian tumors, botryoid sarcoma or carcinoma of the cervix may present similarly. A mucoid vaginal discharge is frequently noted. In the diaper age this is usually due to irritation by the diaper or the powder used in the diaper region. In older children a foul discharge may be due to tight panties, intertrigo, masturbation, pinworms, infection secondary to a foreign body or to allergy. A thin watery discharge is common in girls for two to three years before onset of menstruation.

A very purulent discharge may be due to gonorrhea. Profuse, frothy, foul-smelling pruritic discharges may be due to Trichomonas. White adherent discharge suggests Candida infection.

<u>Foreign bodies</u> are usually palpated by rectal examination. A white practically odorless discharge has no significance. Any discharge significant of disease is usually accompanied by red inflammation in the surrounding vaginal and urethral structures. Urethral caruncle or <u>prolapse</u> of the urethra may be noted.

<u>Adhesions</u> of the labial mucosa may occur. Imperforate hymen may be noted. This may cause hydrocolpos in the young girl, or hematocolpos in the pubertal girl. The labia minora are prominent in the newborn, then atrophy, and are virtually absent until estrogens are produced at adolescence. Adhesions of the labia majora in the newborn may be a congenital malformation or may occur in children with congenital adrenal hyperplasia.

The vaginal area is always inspected, but vaginal palpation is usually omitted by the pediatrician. If performed, vaginal discharge or foreign body, size of uterus, and presence of ovaries should be noted. The normal uterus measures 1-2 cm. and the ovaries 0.5-1 cm. until puberty.

A large clitoris may be noted. This is usually normal, or an isolated physical finding; however, it may indicate adrenal hyperplasia, or any of the conditions associated with precocious puberty. The clitoris may not
develop in adolescent girls with hypopituitarism or gonadal
dysgenesis. The external genitalia grow very little until
adolescence starts.

In the male, note is made if the position of the urethral orifice is not at the tip of the glans: hypospadias
exists if the opening is on the ventral (inferior) surface,
epispadias if on the dorsal surface of the penis. The
nature of the prepuce is also noted, and it is examined
for infection and phimosis, a small opening of the prepuce.
Some adhesions of the prepuce to the glans are normal until about the age of four years. Foreign body may be felt
as a hard mass in the urethra. The prepuce may be inflamed, swollen, and tender. Inflammation of the glans,
balanitis, may cause urinary obstruction.

An enlarged penis may be noted. This occurs in
children with precocious puberty, central nervous system lesions, some testicular tumors or adrenal hyperplasia. In congenital adrenal hyperplasia the penis is
large but the testes are of normal size. The penis may
appear small if it is obscured by fat in fat boys. The
penis is small in adolescent boys with hypopituitarism.

The meatal opening should always be observed.
Stenosis may cause the opening to appear round instead
of slit-like. Ulcers may cause obstruction to urinary
flow. Strength of stream should be noted in both sexes;
decreased stream indicates obstruction.

Next one looks at the scrotum. Normally, the scrotum of a child who is not cold or frightened is loose, and
in it can be felt testes and cords. Anything else in the
scrotum is abnormal. If the scrotum appears large, one
suspects hernia or hydrocele or both together. Often,
especially in premature infants, the scrotal sac appears
small and underdeveloped. One should, however, put his
index finger and thumb together to make an inverted "V,"
about $\frac{1}{2}$ inch above the center of the inguinal ligament, and
gently push toward the scrotum. Somewhere along the in-

guinal canal, a soft mass will be felt. One should then try to push this mass into the scrotum. Once in the scrotum, the mass should be grasped with the thumb and forefinger of the opposite hand. If it can be brought to this position even though it may immediately retract, the mass is normally descended testis. The procedure is repeated on the opposite side. If the mass is palpable in the inguinal canal but cannot be pushed down, or if the testis is not felt, an undescended testis or abdominal testis is suspected. In the older child, one maneuver to bring the testis down is as follows: Have the boy sit in a chair with his heels on the seat, grabbing his knees. The extra abdominal pressure may push the testis into the scrotum. A small, flat, underdeveloped scrotum probably is the most accurate indication of true maldescent, cryptorchism.

The testes are usually about 1 cm. until puberty, then about twice this size. They remain small in children with hypopituitarism. They are enlarged with infection or tumor of the testis, or with precocious puberty, but not with precocious puberty secondary to adrenal hyperplasia. Hard, enlarged testis without pain suggests tumor.

If the penis is normal or small, and the testes are firm and small, in the adolescent, gonadal dysgenesis (Klinefelter's) may be present.

The left testis is usually lower than the right. The opposite may indicate complete situs inversus.

If the scrotum appears large, changes size or enlarges with coughing or crying, place one finger on the external ring and palpate the scrotum. If the mass now in the scrotum feels firm, it is probably normal testis. If something is palpated in addition to the testis and cord, try to determine whether the sensation obtained is that of fluid, gas or solid structure. Try to reduce the mass in the scrotum by pushing the contents back through the external ring. Masses which cannot be reduced include, in addition to normal structures, incarcerated hernia or hydrocele.

Fluid in the scrotum usually indicates the presence of a hydrocele. Hydroceles are found frequently in children under two years of age. Hydroceles are usually not tender and, with closed tunica vaginalis, usually do not change in size when reduction is attempted. Fluid which fluctuates in volume denotes the presence of a patent tunica vaginalis or indirect inguinal hernia.

Next, shine a light through the mass. If the mass (except the testis) transilluminates and is irreducible, fluid is probably present. If the mass does not transilluminate and is irreducible, hernia is probably present. The use of transillumination may be misleading because at times in young children, bowel in a hernial sac may transilluminate.

If there is a bulge in the inguinal canal or a mass in the scrotum which is neither testis nor fluid; or if, on palpation, one gets the sensation of gas (crepitus), the patient has a visible hernia. If, when one tries to push the mass through the external ring, one feels crepitus, this also indicates hernia. Tenderness may be noted. Herniae, in contrast to hydroceles, are usually tender. Next, auscultate over the scrotal sac. Peristaltic sounds help to indicate the presence of a hernia.

Herniae which, in spite of careful manipulation, cannot be reduced, are said to be incarcerated. Herniae which feel swollen or have become gangrenous, are strangulated due to the tight constriction of the neck of the sac.

Finally, if a hernia or hydrocele is suspected, feel over the internal ring with the flat part of the index finger, and roll the spermatic cord beneath the fingers as it lies in the inguinal canal. Though the ring is normally open, a solid structure only should be felt going through the ring. If, in addition to this solid structure, the cord feels thickened or if one gets the sensation of silk being rubbed on silk, peritoneum is going through the ring, denoting a hernia which may be invisible. The size of the structures in the canal can also be determined in this manner, and thickened structures may indicate some abnormality. Occasionally a hydrocele of the spermatic cord can be felt and may be mistaken for a hernia which is incarcerated. Careful palpation of the mass helps to separate the upper end of the hydrocele from the internal ring, which is not possible with a hernia. If the mother reports the presence of a hernia but none is found, the following maneuvers may make the hernia obvious. The infant should be stood on the examining table and the flat of the examiner's hand placed on the abdomen. The abdomen is pumped in and out with several short frequent strokes, and the hernial sac will become apparent. The older child may be sat on a stool and asked to hold his knees while the examiner tries to straighten the legs. The hernial sac will then fill.

Acute swelling of the scrotum with discoloration may be due to torsion of the spermatic cord, a surgical emergency. Acute painful swelling also occurs in boys with orchitis or epididymitis, or rarely torsion of the testis or its appendages. With torsion the testicle is higher in the scrotum than it should be, and may appear to lie transversely. With epididymitis the testicle is in the normal position, and the long axis usually is in the axis of the body. The spermatic cord is tender and swollen with epididymitis, tender but not swollen with torsion. Elevation of the swollen tender mass increases the pain of testicular torsion. Elevation decreases the pain in epididymitis. Epididymitis is usually accompanied by signs of urethral infection. Differential diagnosis of testicular torsion, incarcerated inguinal hernia, epididymitis and orchitis, all of which cause scrotal swelling, may be difficult. Orchitis is usually accompanied by mumps or other viral infection.

The cremasteric reflex is tested by stroking the inner aspect of the thigh. The testis will rise in the scrotum, sometimes going up into the canal. This reflex is normal at any age. Absence may indicate a low spinal cord lesion, as in poliomyelitis; but it is also frequently absent in normal boys, especially below six months and over 12 years.

The lymph nodes in the inguinal region are examined for size and tenderness. Ordinarily three or four 0.5-1.0 cm. glands are not abnormal. Tenderness or enlargement always indicates infection in any area from the feet to the perineum, or any of the systemic diseases associated with generalized enlarged nodes.

ANUS AND RECTUM

The anal region is examined routinely in infants and children. However, rectal examination is not performed in a routine examination, but is reserved for those children with symptoms referable to the lower gastrointestinal tract or those with abdominal pain.

The <u>buttocks</u> are noted for masses and firmness. Masses over the coccygeal area are usually sacrococcygeal tumors. Tufts of hair, meningocele, pilonidal dimple or perianal abscess may be noted easily in this area. If a pilonidal dimple is present, it should be carefully inspected for presence of a sinus. Abscesses may be due to <u>rectal fistula</u>. Therefore, the extent of any rectal fistula <u>should</u> be determined by observation and probing if the full extent of the fistula cannot be visualized.

The buttocks are usually firm, even in advanced malnutrition. However, in cystic fibrosis and celiac syndrome they are flattened. The skin creases of the buttocks are usually asymmetrical, but may indicate the presence of congenitally dislocated hips. Skin creases of the buttocks are especially prominent in children with recent weight loss.

<u>Anal fissure</u> appears as a cut or tear in the mucosa. It is one of the most frequent causes of constipation or rectal bleeding in an infant up to two years of age and may cause infantile "colic." It is best noted by placing the infant on the abdomen, pulling the buttocks apart, and noting the fissure and asymmetry of mucosal folds. Bleeding may occur following this maneuver.

<u>Prolapse</u> of the rectal mucosa is noted. Prolapsed mucosa may be a cause of infantile colic. Prolapse may be caused by chronic constipation or diarrhea, and may occur with cystic fibrosis. Rarely, it is seen in pertussis, and usually it is caused by straining.

<u>Other protrusions</u> from the anus are noted. Small <u>mucosal tabs</u> have no significance. However, cherry-red round protrusions may be rectal <u>polyps</u> and cause rectal bleeding. Solid dark protrusions are <u>hemorrhoids</u> and may be due to portal hypertension. They are rarely found in children. Large flat tabs of the skin may be <u>condylomas</u>, a sign of syphilis.

Occasionally pinworms are noted in the perianal
area in the folds of rectal mucosa, and may cause rectal
itching.

A dark ring around the rectal mucosa may be an
early sign of lead poisoning.

Most of the eruptions around the rectum are due to
diaper rash. Usually, the eruption is a generalized reddened or brawny area with vesicles or papules. However,
pustules may be present and represent secondary infection of the diaper rash or perianal cellulitis due to streptococcus.

A rectal examination is best done with the infant or
child on his back and the legs flexed. If the child is old
enough, he should be asked to empty his bladder before
this examination. Ordinarily, the fifth finger is long
enough to give the required information and hurts the patient less than a larger finger. Because one has better
control and mobility of the index finger, this may be used
for more precise information. The anus and finger cot
are well greased before insertion. Imperforate anus is
noted immediately, as the finger cannot enter beyond the
dimple.

Sphincter tone is noted. A patulous rectum is associated with a low cord injury, including myelomeningocele or diastematomyelia. A tight sphincter is generally
a developmental variation indicating stenosis. Anal stenosis may cause constipation and pain on defecation.

Rectovaginal fistulas are noted by having the finger
enter the vagina.

Occasionally, one feels a shelf-like protuberance
2-5 cm. above the anus. This feeling of a shelf with absence of feces in the rectum may be a sign of aganglionic
megacolon. The anus and rectum may be distended with
feces in children with mental deficiency, chronic constipation, or with psychogenic difficulties. Absence of feces in
the rectum in an acutely ill child may indicate ileus, peritonitis or obstruction.

Masses are noted. Fecal masses of any consistency
can be removed. A tender mass in the lower quadrants
may be found with a low intussusception. A right lower
quadrant mass is occasionally noted with acute appendicitis

or appendiceal abscess, and sometimes with regional ileitis. Polyps may occasionally be felt in the rectum. Masses which displace the rectum forward frequently are teratomas. Other masses described under examination of the abdomen are also noted and have similar significance.

Occasionally, a prostate will be palpated as a flat mass several centimeters up and on the midline anterior wall of the rectum. Any prostate felt larger than 1 cm. before the age of ten years may indicate precocious puberty or congenital adrenal hyperplasia.

Rectal examination is also useful in palpating the uterus. In the pubertal child and occasionally earlier, the ovaries may also be palpated. The uterus is felt as a 1-2 cm. oval mass anterior to the rectum and about 3 or 4 cm. above the symphysis pubis. When the ovaries are palpable, they are about 0.5-1.0 cm. in diameter, about 2-3 cm. lateralward and just above the uterus. Foreign bodies in the vagina or rectum can also be felt by this method.

Even though this examination is usually uncomfortable and is reserved for the last part of the physical, tenderness in the abdomen can frequently be localized by rectal examination. After the finger is well up in the rectum it is placed in the midline, the other hand pressing toward the finger. Facial expression is noted. Next the finger and the abdominal hand are moved to the left; the face is noted; and finally this maneuver is repeated on the right. Differences in facial expression or rigidity of the lower abdomen are clues to abdominal or rectal pathology.

Sensation should be tested in those children in whom a spinal cord lesion is suspected or who have a patulous rectal sphincter. A pin is used to touch the entire perineal region at closely approximated points. Normally, twitching of the perineum occurs with a slight lateral movement of the anus. Absence of this reflex suggests lower motor neuron lesion.

If one desires to visualize the rectal mucosa for suspected internal rectal fissure, polyp or bleeding site, this may be done with relative ease with a small proctoscope or without special equipment. A clean Wassermann tube is greased and pushed about 2 inches into the rectum. A small light is then placed just behind the shoulder and shining into the tube. The tube is slowly withdrawn, and one notes the mucosa as it falls back into place.

CHAPTER VII

Extremities, Spine, Joints and Muscles

In practice, one usually examines the bones, joints and muscles simultaneously. Then, if abnormalities are found, the systems under suspicion are examined individually.

The order of examination of these systems depends largely on the age, condition and cooperation of the child. If the child walks, preliminary observations of posture, gait and stance can be made immediately. The position the child assumes during the examination may be noted either during this part of the examination or as part of the general appearance of the patient.

EXTREMITIES

In the two- to six-year-old age group one may begin the physical examination with observations of the hands and feet. Most children of these ages are happy to show their hands and feet when requested and are especially happy to see no instruments present at the beginning of the examination.

Infants who hold both their arms immobile in 90-degree flexion at the elbow when lying, sitting or standing may be suffering from emotional deprivation. Those infants appearing to look at one arm for a long time or who hold one arm in an unusual position for one or two minutes may have infantile autism. Such posturing is normal up to about six months of age.

Congenital anomalies of the arms, hands, legs and feet are noted. These include amelia (absence of the part), webbing and extra digits.

Length and shape of the extremities are usually de-

termined by nutritional and congenital factors. Abnormalities may sometimes be noted. For example, long
thin extremities are noted in children with arachnodactyly.
Broad short extremities are noted in children with mongolism, gargoylism or chondrodystrophies. Apparent
shortening of the thumb, fourth and fifth fingers occurs
almost always in children with pseudohypoparathyroidism.

Shortening of an extremity is usually congenital, but
may be due to diseases of the epiphyses or cerebral palsy.
Inequality of leg length may be present in children after
femoral fractures, or with dislocation of the hip or other
hip disorders.

Lengthening of an extremity is usually congenital,
but may be due to large hemangiomas, lymphangiomas,
arteriovenous fistula, neurofibromatosis, or hemihypertrophy. Generalized enlargement of the extremities may
occur from any of these factors and when unilateral may
cause hemigigantism. Enlargement may also be due to
congenital lymphedema, Milroy's disease, or as a manifestation of ovarian dysgenesis - Turner's syndrome.

The fingers and toes are noted for clubbing. Elevation of the nail base is an early sign of clubbing. Later,
the entire end of the finger including the nail region seems
expanded and rounded when compared with the remainder
of the finger. Clubbing may occur in any condition of reduced circulating oxygen, such as cyanotic congenital
heart disease or chronic pulmonary disease, and also in
patients with chronic liver disease or bacterial endocarditis.

Pain and tenderness in the extremities are usually
due to trauma or infection. Pain, especially of the legs,
is noted in infants with scurvy. Infants under three months
of age with congenital syphilis may have pain causing
pseudoparalyses. Tenderness over the sartorius muscle
may be noted in children with tuberculous meningitis.
Tenderness elicited at a point in the bone by sharp percussion of the distal end of the bone suggests the presence
of osteomyelitis (Fig. 21).

Pain in the knee or foot may be due to local disease,
but also requires examination of the hips. Pain in the

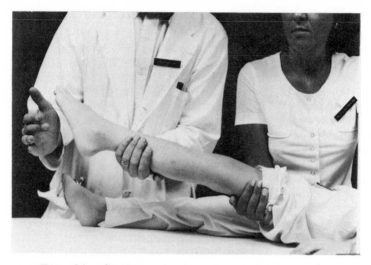

Fig. 21. Striking the foot to elicit pain of osteomyelitis in the tibia or fibula.

knee increased with internal rotation of the tibia may be due to osteochondritis dissecans.

Temperature of the extremities is noted, with special care to note whether the temperature in the extremities is equal. Differences in temperature are usually due to neurological or vascular abnormalities. Cold, pallid extremities may occur following sympathetic nervous system stimulation, or may be a manifestation of venous or arterial thrombosis or embolism. With nervous system lesions, pulsations are usually present, whereas with vascular lesions, pulsations are usually diminished or absent.

Necrosis of the extremity, gangrene, may be noted and is due to obliteration of the vascular supply. The area is cold, avascular, pallid and tender, with loss of muscle power. The area may gradually become black and less painful as necrosis proceeds. It may ooze and be moist and obviously infected, or it may be dry. It may occur in infants following embolism, particularly from the umbilical venous system, following severe trauma or infection to the part, or sometimes following frostbite.

Enlargement of the bones is noted. It may be due to infection in the bone. Swelling with point tenderness, heat and redness near but not in the joint, is characteristic of osteomyelitis. Swelling may be due to periosteal hemorrhage, as in scurvy; to cortical thickening, as in congenital syphilis, vitamin A poisoning, or infantile cortical hyperostosis; to localized increased calcification as in callus formation after fracture, or in rickets; or to bone cysts or tumors. Auscultation over the area of the swelling may reveal a bruit, more common in osteomyelitis than in the other causes of increased vascularity of the bone.

Enlargement of the tibial tubercles with tenderness is characteristic of Osgood-Schlatter disease, probably due to stress on the patellar tendon.

Bony, painless swelling at the epiphysis adjacent to the knee or wrist joints is one of the most definite signs of rickets. Symmetrical swelling of both hands or both feet in infants may indicate the hand-foot syndrome of sickle-cell anemia.

Other deformities of the bones are usually due to fractures. Fractures are noted by the patient's inability to use the limb, by deformity, or by excess motion in the bone with pain and crepitation. Fractures are almost always due to trauma. Multiple fractures may be due to polyostotic fibrous dysplasia, bone cysts, other diseases of the parathyroid gland, prolonged bed rest, or osteogenesis imperfecta.

Shape of the bones is noted. Lateral bowing of the tibia, genu varum, is present when the child stands with the medial malleoli in apposition, and a persistent space of more than one inch is observed between the medial surfaces of the knees. Frequently the infant is bowlegged for one year after starting to walk. Significant genu varum may be due to anomalies of the feet, or to rickets. Anterior curvature of the tibia may indicate congenital syphilis. Excess bowing just below the knee may indicate osteochondrosis deformans, Blount's disease or tibia vara.

Knock-knees, genu valgum, can be determined when, with the knees together, the medial malleoli persistently are separated more than one inch. Knock-knees are usually normal in children from about two to 3-1/2 years of age. Knock-knees may also be seen in children with pronated feet, or with poliomyelitis, rickets, or syphilis.

Bony hard enlargement of the medial or external aspects of the femoral or tibial epiphyses is usually a normal variant but may occur with rickets, other metabolic bone diseases or in dysgenesis of the knees such as dysplasia epiphysealis hemimelica.

Tibial torsion, a twisting of the tibiae probably initiated by intrauterine position, is best determined with the patient on his back and the knees facing upward. Both the forefoot and hindfoot will be held in a plane but not in line with the knees. With the tibial tubercle and the patella in a straight line, the fingers are placed on the malleoli. In an infant, the line joining the four malleoli should be parallel to the table. In the older child, up to 20-degree external torsion is normal. Any greater deviation is considered tibial torsion. With fixed deformities of the foot such as metatarsus varus, the forefoot will be adducted in this position but the hindfoot will be in a straight line with the patella.

The feet are noted for abnormalities. The feet at birth are usually held in varus or valgus attitude, almost never straight. An easy method to determine whether this position, which was the intrauterine position, will straighten is simply to scratch first the outside, then the inside of the lower border of the foot. In self-correctible deformities, the foot will assume a right angle with the leg. More severe anomalies, such as clubfeet or metatarsus varus, can be straightened only with forceful manual stretching, or cannot be straightened by manual means at all.

Since all children have a fat pad under the arch, the feet may appear flat until the child has walked for two years. A very high-arched foot, pes cavus, may be noted in some normal children or may be seen in patients with Friedreich's ataxia, poliomyelitis or various lower motor neuron lesions. Pes equinus, with short heel cords and weight-bearing on the toes, may be a characteristic of children with cerebral palsy or muscular diseases due to spasm and contracture of the muscles of the feet.

The heel cords are examined with the patient supine and his knee extended. The foot is grasped by the heel (Fig. 22), the sole lies in the examiner's hand, and the foot is slightly inverted to lock the heel and then dorsiflexed. Tight cords are present if dorsiflexion cannot be carried to about 20 to 30 degrees beyond a right angle.

Pronation of the feet should be noted. Pronation becomes apparent when the child stands. A pronated foot is flexible and may appear normal when the child lies on the

Fig. 22. Lock heel in palm of hand before testing for tight heel cords.

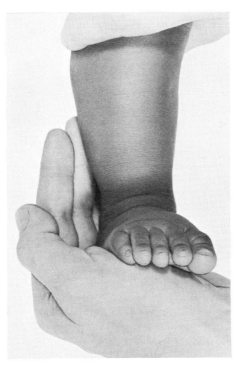

table, but it will abduct at the forefoot when the patient stands, with obliteration of the long arch, bulging of the medial border of the foot, and outward angulation of the forefoot on the hindfoot. The medial malleolus may appear closer to the floor than normal, there may be knock knees, and the thighs may appear adducted. The weight-bearing line, which is the line through the middle of the patella perpendicular to the floor, will cross the inner border of the foot instead of going through the second toe as is normal. From the back, the heel cord, which normally descends perpendicularly, will be noted to curve outward with eversion of the heel (valgus heel).

After examining the feet, the patient's shoes are observed. Abnormal wear or misshapen shoes may help diagnose gait or foot disorders.

The patient's gait and stance are then noted. It is helpful, when studying the child's gait, to observe him in a room with a mirror at one end. The examiner can observe the anterior and posterior aspects simultaneously as the child walks toward and away from the mirror. When observing the child's gait, the child should be wearing shoes or at least socks, as bare feet on a cold floor may distort the gait. Normally, the one- to two-year-old walks with a broad-based gait, frequently with his hands out to the side. Gradually, as the child reaches three or four years, the legs are brought together and the child toes straight ahead. The older child with a broad-based gait may have abnormal mechanics of the legs or feet, or may utilize this gait for balance if his normal neural positioning and balancing mechanisms are defective.

Balance, at rest or while walking, is maintained by normal cerebellar function, normal vestibular nerve function, and good muscle, bone and joint function. Loss of balance may be due to cerebellar or vestibular disease or to muscle weakness. Deviation to one side during walking may indicate cerebellar disease of that side. Lack of normal swing of the arm of that side suggests cerebellar involvement.

Toeing in, pigeon-toe, or toeing out may be noted. Children with pronated feet may toe in or toe out. Other

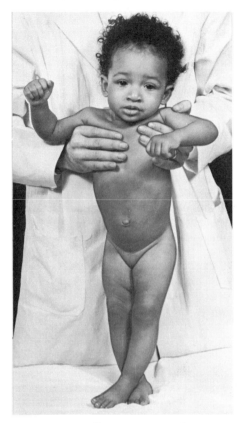

Fig. 23. "Scissors" gait can be demonstrated before child can walk by grasping under axillae and pushing patient forward.

orthopedic conditions causing toeing in include internal rotation of the hips, tibial torsion and metatarsus adductus.

A "scissors" gait with a stiff crossing over of the legs as the child walks, is noted especially in those with a spastic type of cerebral palsy, or with other types of mental deficiency. This type of gait can be elicited even in a seven-month-old if he is made to walk by gripping under his shoulders and pushing him along (Fig. 23). A waddling gait may be noted in patients with bilateral dislocation of the hip, or with coxa vara.

Limp of any type should be noted. Limp may be due
to local infection, muscle, nerve, bone or joint disease,
but it is most commonly due to trauma, fatigue or hip
pathology. Pain in the foot, ankle, knee or hip requires
careful examination of all four, as hip pathology may be
referred to the foot or knee.

Ataxia is noted as gross incoordination. Brain tumors, especially of the cerebellum, and the encephalitides
may be accompanied by ataxia. Ataxia due to sensory or
proprioceptive loss is worse with the eyes closed. The
general weakness characteristic of the amyotonias or
spasm of the muscles of the thigh in hip disease (p. 159)
is sometimes mistaken for ataxia. Other cerebellar injuries, such as cerebral palsy with cerebellar involvement, the degenerative ataxias, some central nervous
system infections or tick paralysis are especially likely
to be followed by ataxia. A variety of drugs, including
Dilantin, phenobarbital, and the antihistamines, may
cause ataxia in sensitive persons. Vestibular damage,
as is sometimes seen in children treated with streptomycin, may be followed by ataxia.

SPINE

The spine should be examined in routine physical examinations. ᐧThe infant is observed while he is lying on
his back. He may kick and move during the examination.
Then he is placed on his abdomen. Observations in the
older child can be made with the patient in the sitting or
standing position.

Tufts of hair, dimples, discolorations, cysts or
masses are frequently seen near the spine. A tuft of hair
over a small dimple in the midline usually indicates the
presence of an underlying spina bifida or may simply be an
ectodermal anomaly. Spina bifida occulta can occasionally
be determined by pressing carefully over the area under
suspicion when the trunk is flexed. The spinous processes
above and below the spina bifida will feel thin and well-
formed while that of the defective vertebra may feel split.

A small dimple in the midline anywhere from the

coccyx to the skull usually indicates a dermoid sinus.
These dimples are important to note as possible entry
points of infection to the central nervous system.

Masses over the spine should be palpated and transilluminated. Non-tender masses of varied color and consistency with a thin covering are usually meningoceles.
Meningoceles, which communicate with the central nervous
system, can usually be distinguished from non-communicating masses by palpation. If signs of increased intracranial pressure, such as bulging of the fontanel, occur,
it is likely that the contents of the mass communicate with
the spinal canal. Cystic masses which transilluminate
may be teratoma, meningocele or lipomeningocele. Non-
tender, non-communicating masses near the spine are
usually lipomas or fibromas. Soft masses feeling like
lipomas, usually with skin dimples, may also extend into
the central nervous system and are lipomeningoceles.
Tender masses not communicating with the spinal canal
are usually infectious and include tuberculous spondylitis
and tuberculous and perinephric abscesses. Deep tenderness over the spine is usually due to trauma of the spine
or surrounding structures. Localized spine tenderness
is best elicited by punching with the side of the hand or by
tapping with the reflex hammer. Localized tenderness
may indicate a cord tumor or injury or infection of an
intervertebral disc.

Masses covered by skin over the sacrum or coccyx
may be teratomas. These are firm and can usually also
be felt on rectal examination.

The spine is examined for intrinsic motion. Limitation of flexion is easily demonstrated by asking the patient
to sit up from a prone position. He turns over and main-
tains the position of his back with poker-like rigidity. If
sitting, the patient is asked to kiss the knees to demonstrate limitation of forward bending. If the fingers of the
examiner are placed on several of the patient's adjoining
spinous processes, normally they will move separately as
the patient bends the trunk laterally. With stiffness of the
spine, the examiner's fingers move as a unit.

The spine is stiff in children with central nervous

system infections, especially poliomyelitis or meningitis,
or with tetanus; with diseases or anomalies of the bones
such as osteomyelitis of the spine, epiphysitis of the vertebrae, or hemivertebrae; or with adjacent lesions such
as peritonitis or perinephric abscesses. Occasionally
with severe trauma to the back, the spine will be rigid.
Such causes of limitation of motion of the spine in adults
as osteoarthritis, protruding intervertebral disc and
lumbosacral strain, almost never occur in childhood.
Severe pain and tenderness over the spine, particularly at
night, may be due to tuberculous abscess or cord tumor.

Limitation of motion of the neck by muscle spasm is
a prime neurological sign of nervous system disease and
is discussed with other lesions of the neck. Non-neurological causes of limitation of motion of the neck include
rheumatoid arthritis of the cervical vertebrae, adjacent
infections such as cervical adenitis and retropharyngeal
abscess, rotatory subluxation of the cervical vertebrae,
fracture of the vertebrae, congenital anomalies of the
cervical vertebrae, especially hemivertebrae, or shortening of the sternocleidomastoid muscle producing torticollis
(wryneck).

Opisthotonos, or hyperextension of the spine, is
noted periodically in all normal infants or in infants with
breath-holding spells. True opisthotonos, which is rigid,
prolonged hyperextension of the spine, usually denotes a
completely decerebrate individual and is observed in those
with severe mental deficiency, kernicterus or severe infections of the central nervous system. This has also
been discussed with the examination of the neck.

Excess mobility of the spine is rare. It is most
easily demonstrated with the patient supine. One hand is
placed beneath the head and the other under the knees. As
the spine is flexed, it feels unusually supple, and the knees
may easily approximate the chin. It occurs with those
states which produce generalized hypotonia, such as mongolism, the amyotonias, or Ehlers-Danlos syndrome, and
is sometimes seen in those small children with acute po-
tassium deficiency.

Winged scapulae may be noted when the lower borders of the scapulae extend out loosely from the back with excess mobility. Mild degrees occur often but marked winging may be due to weakness of the muscles around the scapula. This weakness may occur following injury to the long thoracic nerve, with the muscular dystrophies, or with such congenital anomalies as absence of the clavicle (cleidocranial dysostosis) or high scapula with webbed neck (Sprengel's deformity).

Posture is noted. Lordosis and kyphosis are observed as exaggerations of the normal anteroposterior curvatures of the spine. Lumbar lordosis is normal in children throughout childhood and appears to exist in children with protuberant abdomens. Marked lordosis may be due to rickets, muscular dystrophy or weakness of the abdominal wall. Adolescent round back is seen with chronic poor posture and thoracic epiphysitis.

Kyphosis is a sharp anteroposterior angulation of the spine opposite in direction to lordosis. It is usually due to small or collapsed vertebral bodies and is seen with tuberculosis of the spine, but it may be a diagnostic sign of gargoylism, Morquio's disease or aseptic necrosis of the vertebral bodies. Localized kyphosis, gibbus, is caused by disease of one or two vertebral bodies and may occur with the same disease states causing kyphosis.

Scoliosis, a lateral curvature of the spine, is best detected by having the patient stand erect, marking the tips of the spinous processes with ink, and noting deviation of these ink-spots from a straight line when the patient stands. Structural scoliosis exists when there is a double curvature with rotation (twisting) on the convexity or if the ink-line does not straighten when the patient bends forward or if one hip appears prominent. Mild scoliosis usually has no rotation, straightens in the prone position, and is related to poor postural habits.

Scoliosis in a child under five years of age is usually due to congenital anomalies or to lung or chest pathology. In older children scoliosis may be idiopathic or be due to difference in leg length, hemivertebrae, rickets, poliomyelitis, muscular dystrophies or neurological disorders such as neurofibromatosis. Some curving of the lower spine is noted in children with acute abdominal pathology such as appendicitis or pyelonephritis.

JOINTS

The joints are examined for <u>heat, tenderness, swelling, effusion, redness</u>, and limitation or pain on <u>motion</u>. Redness, heat and tenderness, signs of infection, are noted by observation and palpation. Effusion in the joint, a sign of any type of joint irritation, can be best determined by ballottement of the joint or by tapping on one side of the joint and feeling protrusion on the other side as a fluid wave is elicited. The most common cause in children of tenderness in one joint with limitation of motion but without other physical signs is synovitis of traumatic or non-specific origin.

With the joint extended, try to push fluid from the outer to the medial side of the joint with the flat part of your hand. A bulge of the synovial lining, particularly on the medial side of the knee, indicates <u>effusion</u>. Transillumination helps recognize the presence of fluid.

Swollen, hot joints are seen in children with rheumatoid arthritis, rheumatic fever, allergic, toxic and infectious arthritis, serum sickness, hemarthrosis or osteochondritis. Motion is limited in these conditions, usually because of pain and spasm of the overlying muscles and tendons. Arthritis of rheumatic fever has been noted to respond to aspirin more rapidly than rheumatoid arthritis. Limitation of joint motion without pain may occur as a congenital malformation. Flexion deformities of the fingers and toes are common. Children with multiple congenital dislocations, as in arthrogryposis, may have severe flexion deformities of many joints. Limitation of joint motion is also common in children with various spastic neurological disorders, described in Chapter VIII.

Excess joint motion is demonstrated by hyperflexing or hyperextending the joint. It is usually due to relaxation of the structures surrounding the joint, physiologically, but is exaggerated in children with mongolism, general debility, amyotonia congenita, and Ehlers-Danlos syndrome. Hypermobility of the joints, especially the wrists, is seen in most children with chorea, due to poor muscle tone, and in children with rickets or malnutrition. Hyper-extension of the knees, <u>genu</u> <u>recurvatum</u>, may be due to intrauterine position; or may be noted in children with spina bifida, arthrogryposis, agenesis of the patella, or other malformations.

The <u>hips</u> should be routinely investigated in infants for <u>congenital dislocation</u> or subluxation. With the infant on his back, the legs are flexed at the knees and the ex-aminer attempts internal and external <u>rotation</u> by holding the knees and simultaneously rotating the thighs (Figs. 24 and 25). It is thus easy to see if the rotation is equal on both sides. Unequal rotation usually is due to decreased mobility of one joint. The hips can be abducted and ex-ternally rotated so that the knees touch the table-top in most infants. With unilateral subluxation, abduction is limited on the affected side (Fig. 25). A "click" may be normal or may be a sign of dislocation following this ma-neuver.

Fig. 24.   Internal rotation of the hips.

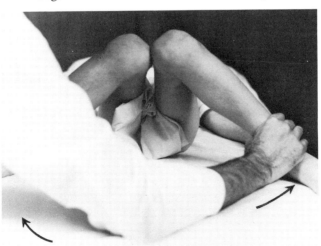

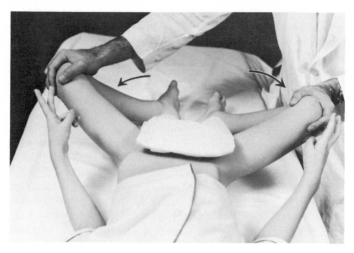

Fig. 25.   External rotation of the hips.   Note that angles made by each leg are equal.

Piston mobility is obtained in children with hip-joint dislocation.   This is determined by holding the hip-region with one hand, grasping the thigh with the other hand, and

Fig. 26.   Piston mobility.   Grasp thigh firmly.

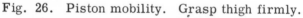

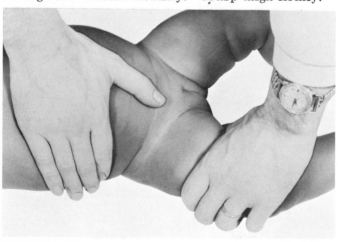

pulling the hands apart gently (Fig. 26).   Motion as occurs in a "Slinky" toy is piston mobility.   A little motion, perhaps up to one-half inch, is normally present; but with congenital dislocation the hip motion may have a range from one inch above to one inch below the socket.   As the child gets older, tightness of the adductor muscles is noted, and the gluteal folds may be uneven.   Uneven gluteal folds may be seen in normal children.

In addition to recognized congenital dislocation, progressive subluxation of the hip may be noted in older children, especially in those who are obese.   The child with dislocation of the hip usually has a painless limp with apparent shortening of the leg on the involved side.   When the child is asked to stand on the normal limb and raise the other leg, the pelvis on the involved side rises to maintain balance.   When the patient is asked to stand on the leg with the dislocated hip and raise the normal limb, the abductor muscles cannot raise the pelvis and it drops (Trendelenburg's sign).   A painless limp, worse with fatigue, occurs also with coxa plana, especially in boys.

All motions of the hip joint may be limited in children with tuberculosis of the hip.   A painful limp, especially in the morning, is usually seen in children with tuberculosis of the hip.   In addition, the hip in this disease is first abducted, and later adducted with flexion on the pelvis.   If it appears that the child is simulating a limp or an abnormal gait, tell him to run, touch a spot, and return. Usually he will concentrate on your instructions and forget to simulate.

MUSCLES

The muscles are noted for development, tenderness, spasm, and paralysis.   Muscle tone is due to a balance between muscle mass and nervous stimulation.   It represents the degree of contraction in the voluntarily relaxed muscle.   Muscle tone is tested by grasping the muscle and estimating its firmness and by watching the muscle response during its normal range of motion with and without resistance, such as response to painful stimuli in the region activated by the muscle.   In the older child muscle

strength is noted by having the child perform the usual
function against resistance supplied by the examiner's
hand.

Muscle tone is decreased in children with general
debility, malnutrition, the dystrophies, some types of
cerebral palsy, lower motor neuron and cerebellar lesions, and many metabolic diseases. It is decreased in
children with poliomyelitis, hypothyroidism, hypopituitarism, mongolism, hypoadrenalism, and hypokalemia.

Muscle tone is increased in any condition causing
muscle spasm. Muscle spasm is felt as unusual tenseness of the muscle mass and may occur with injury or infection of the muscle, bone or joint, with metabolic diseases, or with upper motor neuron lesions. Muscle spasm
is noted also in diseases affecting the spinal cord roots,
probably secondary to pain as in poliomyelitis. Spasm
may occur before pain on occasion as in children with tumors of the cauda equina where hamstring spasm is seen
early.

Generalized spasm may be seen early involving almost all striated muscles in children with tetanus. Spasm
is especially noted with slight disturbances in the environment. The generalized extensor spasm noted with tetanus
may be distinguished from the generalized muscle spasm
of phenothiazine intoxication in that the latter does not
ordinarily involve the abdominal muscles, while in tetanus
the abdomen may be boardlike in its rigidity. Generalized
flexion or extension spasm may be noted in children with
anoxia, and is seen in sickle cell crisis, presumably secondary to local muscle anoxia.

Carpopedal spasm is elicited by restricting the blood
supply to the hand or foot by applying a blood pressure cuff
inflated to the level of the systolic pressure, or by applying a tourniquet or hand around the wrist or ankle for one
or two minutes. Spasm of the muscles of the hands or feet
with marked flexion of the wrists and ankles and extension
of the fingers and toes is then seen. The sign is prominent
especially in children with tetany.

Paresis, weakness or paralysis should be noted.
Paresis generally refers to weakness of a muscle due to

partial paralysis, and the term "paralysis" is usually reserved for complete paralysis. These are demonstrated
by the patient's inability to use a muscle following a command or painful stimulus, or by observing the patient as
he tries to use a particular group of muscles and noting a
lack of motion when certain characteristic movements are
attempted. Paresis and paralysis may be either spastic
or flaccid.

Flaccidity, or flaccid paralysis, refers to the inability of a muscle to maintain its normal tone and position, so that it yields readily and without resistance to
pressure. The muscles in which it occurs should be
noted. Flaccidity usually indicates lower motor neuron
lesion, and occurs in such diseases as poliomyelitis,
amyotonia congenita, myasthenia, tick paralysis or spinal
cord injury. The proximal muscles are usually affected
first in the muscle dystrophies of adults, while primary
neurological disease first affects the distal muscles. This
distinction is not so clear in children. A child who rises
from the supine position by climbing up himself instead of
jumping up may have proximal muscle weakness of the
pelvic muscles. Likewise, he will push himself up to get
out of a chair. Strength in the shoulder girdle can be tested
by lifting the child under the axillae. If the shoulder muscles are weak, the child will slip through the examiner's
arms. Flaccidity may be due to damage of a small area
of the cerebral cortex or of the lateral hemispheres of the
cerebellum; these lesions occur rarely in childhood. It is
noteworthy that, as in adults with brain injury, the paralysis following the upper motor neuron lesion is first flaccid
and later spastic; so also in newborns with brain damage,
the child may be flaccid for as long as six months before
spasticity becomes fixed.

Paresis may also occur with chronic wasting disease,
congenital heart disease, rickets, and other forms of malnutrition. Mild paresis may be noted in children with hyperthyroidism. Normally a child can hold his leg extended on
command for about one minute, a child with hyperthyroidism about 10 seconds. Unilateral flaccidity may be noted
in children with hemichorea. The leg withdraws on pinprick,

distinguishing this from true paralysis. Paralysis without other neurological signs may be due to hysteria.

In older children and adults proximal weakness occurs more frequently in muscle diseases, and distal weakness in neuropathic diseases. In infants weakness is usually proximal in both myopathies and neuropathies. In children with polyneuritis the proximal muscles are weaker in the legs and the distal muscles in the arms. In children with pyramidal lesions weakness in flexion is greater than that of extension in the legs, but weakness of extension is greater than that of flexion in the arms.

Spasticity refers to a prolonged and steady contraction of the muscle. It is demonstrated by increased resistance to passive movement, and gives way suddenly when overcome — "clasp-knife" rigidity. It is accompanied by increased reflexes and clonus. The muscles are noted in which it exists. Spasticity of a limb occurs with any upper motor neuron disease or following a prolonged painful stimulus. Spasticity is also marked in children with the degenerative brain diseases discussed with muscle spasm. Spasticity of the extensor muscles of the legs, or exaggeration of the postural reflexes, with flexor spasticity in the upper extremities, is more marked in children with brain damage limited to the motor cortex, whereas spasticity of the extensors of both the arms and legs usually indicates more extensive damage in the cortex and the basal ganglia. Spasticity largely of the lower extremities as in spastic diplegia thus is usually accompanied by better mental development.

Rigidity refers to an absolute inability to flex a joint, and is noted in diseases in which there is fusion of the joint. Rigidity of the neck is also noted in children with meningitis and other lesions mentioned in the discussion of the neck. Rigidity of the spine is noted in children with meningitis, poliomyelitis and other lesions discussed with examination of the spine. Usually, the tendon reflexes are absent due to the excessive rigidity.

Cogwheel rigidity of the leg muscles, manifested by spasm followed by weakness after flexion, is characteristic of children with myotonia congenita, Thomsen's dis-

ease. Good strength in the quadriceps muscles rapidly
followed by weakness is noted in children with hyperthyroidism. A strong hand-grip followed by weakness is
seen especially in children with chorea.

Contractures are observed as fixed deformities of
the muscle, with limitation of joint motion, frequently accompanied by muscle atrophy. Contractures may occur
in any state causing continuous spasm or disease of the
muscle.

Muscle atrophy is best determined by either noting
an obvious decrease in muscle mass or, preferably, by
measuring the muscle area and comparing with the opposite side. The latter can be done on the extremities,
but care must be taken that the area measured be exactly
the same bilaterally. For example, if one suspects atrophy of the calf muscles of one side, the circumference of
the calf should be measured on both sides, exactly the
same distance below the knee or above the malleoli.

Muscle atrophy may occur following prolonged spasm
or disuse from any cause including immobilization, malnutrition, joint disease, nervous system lesion and the
muscular dystrophies. Fasciculations of the muscles are
noted as brief repetitive twitches in muscles at rest, and
increased by movement of or pressure on the muscle.
Fasciculations can be augmented by the administration of
neostigmine, 1.0 mg., and atropine, 0.6 mg. They are
usually noted in progressive lower motor neuron disease,
but not myopathy.

Facial myokymia, spontaneous undulating waves of
contracting muscle fibers spreading across facial muscles,
appears most commonly with multiple sclerosis and intra-
medullary pontine tumors.

Muscle hypertrophy is recognized as enlarged musculature with good tone. It usually is compensatory, and
other muscles are found to be atrophic. It may result
from normal exercise or from constant activity, as in
choreo-athetosis. In pseudohypertrophy the muscle appears
large because of fatty infiltration; such muscles are weak.

Muscle percussion is useful in distinguishing myopathy
from lower motor neuron disease. Tap the deltoid, quad-

riceps or gastrocnemius belly briskly.   Normally the muscle contracts.   Response is usually normal in children with neuropathies, but absent in those with myopathies.

CHAPTER VIII

Neurological Examination

As mentioned earlier, the neuropsychiatric examination is one of the most important parts of the examination of the child who is not acutely ill. Since the central
nervous system is one of the most common sites of infection in the infant, this type of examination is also important in the acutely ill infant. It should be remembered
that in addition to careful observation and a careful neurological examination, a detailed history of the child's
development and behavior are necessary for the neurological evaluation.

In addition to an evaluation of the child's development and behavior, the neurological examination of the
child differs from that of the adult in that the neurological lesions usually sought in the child differ from those
in the adult. For example, in children poisonings, congenital malformations of the brain, progressive brain
diseases, and infections are common, whereas local
vascular lesions are rare. Acute brain injury may be
present in both children and adults, but bleeding in children's brains may be accompanied by delayed onset of
signs because of the distensibility of the skull. In children as in adults, metabolic diseases may also often give
central nervous system signs.

This part of the examination should be performed,
except for such overall procedures as the mass reflexes,
with the examination of each particular part of the body.
Listed here are only the mass reflexes, the reflexes found
in the extremities, and general aspects of the neurological examination. However, the neurological examination
may be repeated as a whole after the general physical examination, especially if any variants from the normal are

found or if neurological difficulties are suspected, and may be recorded separately.

More important than the examination of reflexes, except in the child who is acutely ill with a neurological disorder, is the general impression the examiner gets of the patient's abilities and responsiveness.

While older children and adolescents may be examined in a manner similar to that used for adults, the infant and younger child are examined neurologically largely by observation of the characteristic positions of the patient, his spontaneous movements, and his play activity. Some of these qualities have already been discussed in Chapter III, General Appearance. One must utilize imagination and patience in his approach to the patient to elicit this type of information. Especially in infancy, motor and social accomplishments should be compared with suitable developmental charts which, with full realization of the wide variability of normals, help indicate neurological adequacy (Appendix II).

The state of consciousness is noted. The patient may be hyperirritable, convulsive, hyporeactive, delirious, stuporous or comatose. State of consciousness may be difficult to quantitate. Response to commands, speech, name, pinprick or severe pain are some of the usual tests for degree of consciousness, and lack of response in the above order indicates decreasing consciousness and increasing stupor or coma.

Generalized hyperirritability in a child is usually a sign of psychological difficulty. This can frequently be elicited by observing the patient make quick movements if he is asked, for example, to draw a picture. Irritability may, however, be prominent in any child with an acute febrile illness, other disease states such as acrodynia or scurvy, or may indicate central nervous system disorders. Hyperactivity also occurs in children with chorea or hyperthyroidism, hypocalcemia, and other metabolic disorders. Ordinarily, the younger child will be more irritable when lying on the bed or examining table than when in his mother's arms due to a natural fear of the unnatural surroundings. Some infants will be noted to be more irritable when in the mother's arms. This paradoxical irritability should alert the examiner to the possibility of central nervous system infections, particularly meningitis, though other disease states such as acrodynia, scurvy, severe febrile illness, fractures, or emotional disturbances may also manifest this sign.

Convulsive states are signs of disease and should never be considered diagnoses. Seizures manifest themselves in different ways. The type of seizure, the parts of the body involved, and the duration should be recorded. Major seizures may be observed as generalized, completely incoordinated, tonic and clonic movements in unconscious children and are due to abnormal cortical discharges. Petit mal seizures are brain disturbances causing loss of consciousness for 5 to 15 seconds and are also accompanied by abnormal electrical brain discharges. Psychomotor seizures may be characterized by alterations in consciousness and abnormal motor activity; autonomic seizures may consist of bizarre visceral disturbances. Most childhood seizures begin on one side and may be thought to be focal, but quickly become generalized and the etiology is usually that of a generalized seizure. All types of seizures are probably caused by cortical or subcortical irritability. The causes of the irritability may include many types of metabolic, vascular or central nervous system disorders. Seizures do not usually occur in children with brain tumors until the intracranial pressure is considerably elevated. Seizures should be distinguished from simple fainting, syncope, which is sudden loss of consciousness without abnormal movements, usually caused by reflex vascular disorders or hysterical fits which are usually not accompanied by injuries or other neurological signs. Seizures preceded by crying or cyanosis are commonly associated with breath-holding spells. Opisthotonos is more common with breath holding. Syncopal episodes occur suddenly, but with premonitory sensation occur more commonly when the child is sitting, standing, or coughing. Seizures can occur when the patient is lying down.

Lack of gross activity, demonstrated by the persist-

ence of one position for long periods of time, is common
in mentally or emotionally retarded children or may be a
sign of severe debility, malnutrition or anemia. Cata-
tonia, in which one unusual or apparently uncomfortable
position is assumed for a long time, may be seen in mentally retarded or psychotic children. Catatonia-like observation of the fingers and hands is normal in the three-
to six-month-old child.

Lack of all activity is usually due to a state of unconsciousness - stupor or coma - and must be differenti-
ated from normal sleep states from which the patient can
be easily aroused. Unconsciousness in children may be
due to many types of central nervous system lesions,
metabolic abnormalities or poisoning.

In the older child who can walk, other neurological
evaluations are made before the reflexes are elicited. The
patient's gait, stance, limp or ataxia are noted; they have
been described in Chapter VII.

Incoordination is noted. Incoordination may be
caused by cerebellar lesions or by any of the diseases
which may cause ataxia. Watch the child reach for a toy,
tear paper, tie shoes or button his shirt. Coordination is
easily tested by playing a game with the child. The examiner sits opposite the child with his palms upward and asks
the child to strike first the examiner's right, then left hand.
This continues at a rapid pace and the examiner then shifts
the position of his hands. Inability of the child to follow
the motion of the examiner's hands may indicate varying
degrees of incoordination.

Coordination may also be tested by the finger-to-
nose or heel-to-shin tests in the child who can understand
commands. In these tests, the patient is told to extend
first one hand and touch the tip of his nose with the index
finger. This is then repeated with the opposite hand, usually after a demonstration by the examiner. The test is
then repeated after the patient is told to do the same procedure with his eyes shut. Gross incoordination will be
noted as the failure of the patient to touch his nose with
his eyes open. Minor evidences of incoordination, as
well as lack of sense of position, will be manifested by
the patient's inability to perform these tests with his eyes

shut. It should be remembered that fine coordination is not fully developed in children until four or even six years of age and, if the younger patient can bring his finger within one or two inches of the tip of the nose, this is generally considered normal.

The heel-to-shin test is performed by telling the patient to run the heel of one foot down the anterior aspect of the tibia of the other foot. Usually, the examiner also demonstrates this to the patient. Inability to perform this test is a less reliable guide to evidences of incoordination or lack of position-sense in a child, but tests with the eyes open and shut are similar in significance to those of the finger-to-nose test. Romberg's sign, discussed later, is also a test of sense of position.

Tremors are noted and distinguished from choreiform movements. Tremors are constant small movements; some occur when the patient is at rest due to lesions of the extrapyramidal system, and some occur only when voluntary motion of the part is attempted (intention tremor). Intention tremors are due to lesions of the cerebellum. Tremors in the young infant are seen with states of hypocalcemia and hypoglycemia. Muscular tremors or fibrillations may be noted when certain muscles are fatigued and may also be noted in children with hyperthyroidism, hypothermia, hyperthermia or progressive nervous degeneration of the cord. Most commonly, however, tremors or twitchings may occur in infants in bursts, without obvious cause.

Twitchings or spasmodic movements of short duration, are noted in fatigued muscles, in muscles in which a nerve is regenerating, or in chorea. Twitchings may occur following sharp pain to an area. Twitchings also occur in emotionally upset children, follow a definite and usually periodic pattern, and are due to habit spasm.

Choreiform movements are coarse, involuntary, purposeless movements associated with decreased muscle tone. They are quick, jerky and irregular movements, grossly incoordinated, and may disappear with relaxation. In chorea, they may include the muscles of the tongue, speech muscles, the muscles of the hands and feet or any other muscles. These movements are best elicited by

having the patient extend his hand or perform other voluntary acts. The fingers and wrists hyperextend and the
choreiform movements of the fingers become exaggerated.
With extension of the arms above the head, the palms of
the hand point outward and the hand is flexed at the wrist
with extension of metacarpal and interphalangeal joints.
Choreiform movements are also noted in patients with hereditary ataxias. Choreiform movements may be one-
sided, hemichorea, or rarely may be due to vascular brain
lesions, hemiballism.

Athetosis refers to a group of constant gross incoordinated movements which are slow, writhing, and usually associated with increased muscle tone. These movements are exaggerated by voluntary activity. The movements disappear when the patient relaxes during sleep.
Dystonia is a slow twisting movement of limbs or trunk.
Athetosis usually indicates deep central nervous system,
basal ganglia, involvement; ataxia and incoordination occur with even superficial cerebellar lesions. Athetoid
movements may occur in children with cerebral palsy,
tuberous sclerosis, and late in the downward course of
the reticuloendothelial diseases such as Niemann-Pick
and Tay-Sachs. Infants normally may have athetotic movements during their first year. A periodic nodding of the
head, spasmus nutans, resembles athetosis. It may be
idiopathic, may occur as a habit spasm or may be a sign
of mental deficiency. The nodding is a combination of true
anteroposterior nodding and lateral shaking which may be
temporarily interrupted by suddenly attracting the child's
attention. Infants with spasmus nutans usually also tilt
the head and have nystagmus. To-and-fro motions of the
head synchronous with the pulse, de Musset's sign, may
occur with aortic insufficiency.

Associated movements, or voluntary movement of
one muscle accompanied by involuntary movement of
another muscle, are noted. These movements are reg-
ulated by the cerebellum. They occur as mirror movements in the Klippel-Feil syndrome, in diseases with increased intracranial pressure, and in patients whose
handedness has been changed. Reciprocal movements

occur normally in infants two to four months of age and usually decrease by four to six months; failure of these movements to appear or disappear at the proper times are an indication of brain damage. Certain reciprocal movements, such as the movement of the arms when a person walks, are normal at all ages and their absence may indicate cerebellar damage.

Rigidity, spasticity, pareses, and paralysis should be noted. They are described in Chapter VII. Handedness should be noted by observing the preferential handling of small objects. Definite handedness in a child less than 15 months suggests hemiparesis.

The superficial reflexes are the abdominals, the cremasterics, and the skin reflex of the anus, which have been discussed. Reflexes may be reinforced by having the child grasp the examiner's hand or by moving other parts of his body.

The deep tendon reflexes of the extremities are obtained by briskly tapping the biceps, triceps, patella, and Achilles tendons with the flat of the finger. Usually, a hammer or stick should be used only in the older child. The child should relax or the physician should talk to him or otherwise catch him unawares or casually, to best elicit these reflexes. The muscle to be stimulated should be able to act at maximal mechanical advantage; usually this is a position of about half flexion of the joint involved. Examination of these reflexes, though easy to obtain and rarely forgotten, are only a small part of the neurological examination of the child. Tendon reflexes are stretch reflexes and are elicited by a rapid stretch of the muscle. They are elicited only in the presence of intact sensory nerves from the muscle to the spinal cord, intact nerves in the spinal cord, and intact motor nerves from the cord to the muscle. The knee jerk is usually present at birth and is followed by the Achilles and brachial reflexes. The triceps reflex should be present at six months.

Hyperactivity of the deep tendon reflexes indicates upper motor neuron lesion, hyperthyroidism, hypocalcemia, or brain stem tumor. Hyperactivity of the deep tendon reflexes may also occur in areas of muscle spasm,

such as early poliomyelitis. Diminution or absence of
these reflexes is found in the amyotonic or myasthenic
muscular dystrophies or lower motor neuron lesions, including polyneuropathy. Patients with cerebellar tumors
usually have decreased reflexes. Knee reflexes may be
lost early in diphtheria, later in poliomyelitis. Decreased
reflexes are frequently associated with flaccidity or flaccid
paralysis. Flaccidity associated with active reflexes may
be seen in children with some forms of brain injury, mongolism, malnutrition, and some disorders of amino acid
metabolism. A normal contraction with delayed relaxation of the knee and ankle jerks may occur in children with
hypothyroidism. Progressive extension of the leg on suc-
cessive tapping of the patellar tendon, due to failure of the
leg to return to the resting position, occurs in chorea
(pendular knee jerk).

Clonus is a series of forced alternating contractions
and partial relaxations of the same muscle. It may be
demonstrated as a persistence of a rhythmic reflex after
the stimulus, such as striking the tendon with a hammer,
has been withdrawn; ordinarily, a reflex exhausts itself
for a few seconds after it is once obtained. If the clonus
occurs without further stimulation, it is said to be sus-
tained. If repeated stimulation is necessary, it is unsus-
tained.

Clonus of the knee is most easily obtained with the
lower leg swinging freely over the bed or examining table
while the patient is in the sitting position. The patellar
tendon reflex is elicited in the usual manner, a hyperactive
knee-jerk is usually obtained, and clonus exists if the patella or the muscles around the knee-joint continue to con-
tract and relax, causing the lower leg to jerk forward and
back repeatedly. Clonus of the knee may also be obtained
if the knee is flexed, the leg above the knee is grasped with
one hand, the leg below the knee is grasped with the other
hand, and the lower hand of the examiner is pushed quickly
against his upper hand. The rapid contractions or relaxations will either be felt or seen.

Clonus of the ankle is best obtained by having the
child lie down, with the knee flexed slightly, and the ankle
resting comfortably with the toes pointing outward and up-

ward. With the left hand the lower ankle is lightly held and the second finger of the right hand or the hammer taps the tendon. Either the reflex or the clonic movement is felt in the left hand. If clonus is not elicited, the leg is placed flat on the table with the toes pointing upward; the ankle is flexed quickly. Clonus is felt in the hand causing the flexion.

Clonus is an exaggeration of hyperactive deep tendon reflexes. It may occur with fatigue but frequently indicates any of the diseases causing hyperactive reflexes. Taken as a group, increased muscle tone, increased tendon reflexes, clonus, spasticity, rigidity and abnormal pyramidal tract signs described below are indications that point to upper motor neuron lesions, though all these signs may be seen in some metabolic disorders.

Myoclonic jerks are brief involuntary contractures of muscles. Myoclonic seizures are sometimes called infantile spasms, usually represent severe central nervous system disorders, and may be an early sign of tuberous sclerosis.

In the infant under five months of age, the Moro reflex is extremely informative. This is elicited by startling the patient -- either by a loud noise, dropping the patient, or otherwise surprising him. Normally the child reacts as if he is grasping a tree: his arms first extend, then flex; his hands clench, and his knees and hips flex.

Absence of Moro reflex in a newborn infant indicates severe central nervous system injury or deficiency. Persistent Moro reflex after five months of age has the same significance. Absence of Moro reflex of one arm indicates fractured humerus, brachial nerve palsy or recently fractured clavicle. Absence of or irregular Moro reflex of one leg indicates lower spinal injury, myelomeningocele, avulsion of the cord or dislocated hip. Hyperactive Moro reflex indicates tetany, tetanus or central nervous system infection.

A "reverse" Moro reflex consists of extending and externally rotating the arms, with rigidity following the usual stimulus. Such a reflex is seen in children over five days of age who have basal ganglia disease, including kernicterus of erythroblastosis fetalis. Such children may have no Moro reflex within the first five days of life.

The method of eliciting and the significance of the tonic neck reflex have been described.

The Landau reflex is elicited by supporting the infant horizontally in the prone position. The infant raises his head and arches his back. This is normally elicited from 3 months to $1\frac{1}{2}$ years. It represents a combination of labyrinth, neck and visual reactions; its absence suggests motor weakness, upper motor neuron disease or mental retardation.

The Babinski reflex is obtained by scratching the sole of the feet with something such as a broken pointed tongue depressor. Normally the small toes do not move and the great toe moves plantarwise. Abnormally the toes fan out and the great toe moves dorsally. The "abnormal" form is found in most normal children under 18 months of age. Persistence beyond the age of two to two and a half years indicates pyramidal tract lesion. Sometimes one may find it difficult to decide whether the Babinski reflex is present or absent, as only part of the response will be obtained. In such cases, one must look for other signs of upper motor neuron lesions before concluding that the response is abnormal. Oppenheim's sign is obtained by pressing on the median aspect of the ankle and noting the toes as in Babinski's sign. The significance is the same. Hoffmann's sign is obtained by snapping the terminal digit of the second finger and noting flexion of the first and third fingers. It, too, usually indicates a pyramidal tract lesion, but is also obtained in children with tetany.

Kernig's sign is the inability to extend the leg with the hip flexed. This sign indicates irritation of the meninges, or hamstring spasm, as in poliomyelitis. This is a difficult sign to evaluate in infants under six months of age.

Romberg's sign is obtained by having the patient stand with his heels together and his eyes shut. Normally, the patient is able to stand without falling. The sign is said to be positive if the child leans toward or falls toward one side. It occurs in children with poor or absent sense of position. It is found in patients with vestibular

damage and cerebellar tumors. The sign is also noted
in children with the cerebellar ataxias.

Foerster's symptom is obtained in children with
generalized hypotonicity. Such children are sometimes
called "floppy infants." The child is raised by his armpits.
The legs straighten as the child is raised if the hypotonia
is due to diseases with paralytic weakness such as the
Werdnig-Hoffmann syndrome or benign variants of it; the
congenital myopathies: nemaline, central core, and others;
metabolic, e.g. glycogenoses, rickets, or the muscular
dystrophies; or other central nervous system disorders,
the hypotonia-obesity syndrome of Prader-Willi, connective tissue diseases, or acute illnesses. If the hypotonia
is due to atonic spastic diplegia, the knees and hips remain
flexed.

Trousseau's sign is obtained by obstructing the
blood flow at the wrist or ankle by making a ring around
the area with the thumb and index finger, or by using the
blood pressure cuff. After three minutes, carpal or pedal
spasm is produced. This sign is present in children with
tetany, hyperirritability or hyperventilation. The peroneal
sign is obtained by tapping the lateral surface of the fibula
just below the head, and noting dorsiflexion and abduction
of the foot. It, also, is seen in children with diseases of
hyperirritability. These signs, in contrast to Chvostek's
sign described with the examination of the face, can be
obtained even in a crying child and may be very helpful in
diagnosing hypocalcemia.

The grasp reflex is obtained by placing a small object in contact with the infant's fingers. He will grasp
the object tightly with his fingers. This movement is
normally present from one month to three months of age.
If absent, brain or local nerve or muscle injury should
be suspected. Presence after four months suggests a frontal lobe lesion. With injury to the brachial plexus, the
fingers may be constantly maintained (spasticity) in the
grasping position or may be flaccid. The hands are normally held as a fist for the first three months of life, then
begin to be held open for longer periods. At about six
months of age the normal infant should begin to take objects with one hand; at about seven months, he should be

able to transfer objects from one hand to the other. After nine months of age, the child should grasp with his fingers and appose the fingers with his thumb, and at 10 months he should develop purposeful release. These responses are delayed in children with mental deficiency or with lesions of the pyramidal tract.

The <u>thumb position</u> itself is important in determining neurological lesions in infancy. The normal thumb position in infancy is in the fist in a straight line with the index finger, or is freely movable in the palm of the hand. The thumb may be forcibly adducted in the palm of the hand in infants with upper motor neuron lesions.

Overall <u>developmental motor activity</u> should be noted. Delayed appearance of normal motor activity may be due to brain damage, peripheral motor damage, emotional or mental retardation, parental neglect or lack of challenge to the infant, prolonged illnesses or anemia.

The one-month-old should be able to support his head for an instant. By four months of age he should be able to hold his head up well and to roll from the supine to the prone position. At about six or seven months he begins to sit and is able to roll over completely. At about nine months of age he creeps and about one year stands with support. He walks at about 14 months, runs stiffly at about 18 months and well at about two years. He usually cannot skip or throw a ball overhand well until about four years of age. For estimation of level of overall developmental motor activity, suitable charts or books of growth and development should be consulted. The importance of the head and chest circumferences, neck and spine mobility, and the status of the fontanels as part of the neurological examination are discussed in Chapter IV. A convenient table for following the developmental progress of infants has been systematized and should become part of each infant's record (Appendix II).

<u>Sensory</u> changes are difficult to determine in childhood because of lack of cooperation. Of the cranial nerves, smell and taste are almost never tested. Blindness and deafness have been discussed. Of the peripheral nerves, testing is almost entirely limited to the perception of pain in the infant. Pain sensation is normal in children with

muscle diseases, and altered in some with neuropathies.

Withdrawal reflexes, which are obtained by applying a mildly painful stimulus and observing an unusually rapid withdrawal, usually indicate hyperesthesia and may be evidence of extensive lesions in the spinal cord. Hyperesthesia is noted early in children with infectious diseases of the central nervous system, diseases with increased intracranial pressure, peritonitis, herpes zoster, and often with many other diseases. Decreased sensation may be noted in children with cord or peripheral nerve lesions, mental deficiency, decreased consciousness, or such unusual states as familial autonomic dysfunction, ectodermal dysplasia and congenital indifference to pain. When an infant is held erect with soles flat on a table-top, he will take regular alternating steps, the stepping reflex. Similarly when prone on a table-top with head erect, he will make crawling movements. These reflex movements should disappear at about five months.

In the child six years of age or older, other sensory responses may be obtained as in adults. Sense of position has been described above with coordination. Vibratory sensations can be tested with a tuning fork. Astereognosis may be determined by asking the child to identify coins or other familiar objects when his eyes are shut. Temperature sensation may be tested by asking the patient which end of the reflex hammer is cooler, when his eyes are shut. The rubber end is usually warmer than the metal end. Cotton may be used to determine areas of decreased sensation to touch. Loss of any or all of these modalities of sensation may be due to mental deficiency or other types of decreased states of consciousness. In the absence of these, abnormal sensory response usually indicates posterior spinal cord root or peripheral nerve lesions or it may be due to emotional disturbances.

The other cranial nerves may be tested as a group proceeding from I to XII. Method of testing response has already been detailed with examination of the head and neck, Chapter IV.

Other non-neurological measurements, such as the character of the pulse, respiration and blood pressure may again be noted here as part of the central control of these functions.

Respirations are shallow and irregular with respiratory center involvement. The pulse is weak, rapid and irregular, the skin is flushed, and the blood pressure is elevated (but may fall later) with circulatory center involvement. Not only infections and mass lesions cause involvement of the cranial centers, but also drugs, poisons, acidosis, alkalosis and water balance may affect these centers.

Finally, note is made of total response of the child, including cooperation, backwardness, lethargy, reaction to physician and parent, etc. These may be recorded in the first statement of one's write-up of general appearance. Special characteristics of mental development may be recorded here.

CHAPTER IX

Examination
of the Newborn

The baby figure
of the giant mass
Of things to come.

(Troilus and Cressida,
Act I, Sc. 3, Shakespeare.)

Though the newborn is a complete individual, a few
special notes are made in his examination. Again, the
question one wants answered is: "Is he normal?" Even
minor abnormalities should be explained to the mother to
allay her fears. In the apparently well infant a second
physical examination should be completed after the infant
has adjusted to his new environment, as some physical
abnormalities may become apparent after several days of
life. However, here one is restricted to gross physical
anomalies and the examination is therefore simpler. One
should have an exact idea of what he wants to know, proceed with the examination expeditiously, and write it up if
even on a check-sheet. There is little need to worry about
patient cooperation as this is non-existent. The baby should
be kept warm, and a sugar-nipple may quiet him for a
short time. If the patient is not crying, it is best to listen
to the chest first. Otherwise, proceed systematically
from the head downward. In general, the first examination of the newborn is an examination chiefly of orifices,
but the actual method of examination is similar to that
already described.

GENERAL

The color and breathing of the baby should be noted.

179

If the baby is gray or cyanotic, or if the respirations are labored, examination should not begin until the airway is gently but rapidly cleared, oxygen has been given and respiration has become regular. If, in the process of clearing the airway of mucus and amniotic fluid, a soft no. 8 feeding catheter with suction is passed first through the nares into the nasopharynx and then down the esophagus to the stomach, and no obstruction is met, the diagnosis of choanal atresia or esophageal atresia, other nasopharyngeal anomalies such as nasal cysts, encephaloceles or tumors can be eliminated. The catheter should be passed swiftly and gently without jerking, lest laryngospasm be induced. The tip of the catheter will be seen or felt throughout the left half of the abdominal wall. If the catheter is not palpable, cardiospasm may be present.
If the catheter is down but not palpable, hold the hand over the abdomen and blow a quick puff of air through the catheter. The air bubble will be felt. If obstruction is met or the bubble is not felt, atresia in either of these areas must be considered as a possible cause of the infant's respiratory difficulty. Auscultating over the stomach while blowing air in may be deceptive, because transmitted sounds may be heard even though obstruction is present.

With the catheter in the stomach, aspirate the gastric fluid. Note the amount and quality. Normal amniotic fluid measures 5-25 cc. and is cloudy white. Bloody fluid suggests placenta previa. Green fluid suggests meconium-stained amniotic fluid due to antepartum asphyxia. More than 25 cc. of fluid suggests gastrointestinal tract obstruction.

Shock in a newborn infant usually is due to heavy sedation of the mother prior to delivery or to intracranial trauma, but it may also be due to generalized trauma of delivery, placental bleeding, a ruptured viscus, or hemorrhage in the adrenal area.

A helpful evaluation of the baby at one minute and at five minutes of life is the Apgar score, the baby's first report card. Five criteria are noted, and each is given 0, 1 or 2 points:

Criterion	Score		
	2	1	0
Heart rate	100-140	100	0
Breathing and cry	prompt lusty	fair	apnea 1-2 gasps
Reflex irritability	good	fair	0
Muscle tone	good	fair or increased	flaccid
Color	pink	fair	blue

A score of 8-10 is excellent, 4-7 guarded, and 0-3 critical.

Gross anomalies such as anencephaly, omphalocele, exstrophy of the bladder or amelia are immediately obvious and will not be discussed. They are, of course, recorded in as much detail as possible.

SKIN

In the systematic examination of the infant, skin color, consistency and hydration are noted.

Normally, soon after birth the infant becomes pink and cries lustily. Cyanosis in the newborn is produced by the same biochemical factors as in the older child. Because the newborn usually has a higher hemoglobin level than the older child, cyanosis occurs more easily and with less relative oxygen unsaturation than in an older child. Occasionally, ecchymoses will be confused with cyanosis. Pressure on a cyanotic area will blanch the skin temporarily; the ecchymotic area remains blue with pressure. Mongolian spots are usually easily distinguished from cyanosis, especially by their location.

An infant who remains cyanotic may have amniotic fluid, stomach contents, or tumors of the tongue or about the mouth obstructing his airway. Persistent cyanosis indicates central nervous system, heart or lung disease

and differentiating between these at an early age is difficult. Cyanosis in an infant with a slow cardiac or respiratory rate, with a bulging fontanel, or with limpness
especially after a rapid delivery (or of a mother who has
been heavily sedated), suggests intracranial injury of the
baby. Cyanosis with shock may occur because of poor
perfusion, such as with a perforated viscus or septicemia.

Cyanosis which lessens when the infant cries, especially if he is in a high oxygen atmosphere, suggests
the presence of pulmonary disease, especially atelectasis.
That cyanosis which increases when the infant cries suggests cardiac disease. This test of the influence of crying
on the depth of cyanosis distinguishes that due only to heart
or lung disease and crying should not be induced in any infant suspected of having brain injury as the increased intracranial pressure caused by crying may aggravate intracranial hemorrhage.

Localized cyanosis which may persist for 24-48 hours
may sometimes be noted in a presenting part. Usually, if
a normal baby is slightly cyanotic at birth, cyanosis will
be less in the hands than in the feet after about four hours
of age. Equal cyanosis in the hands and feet after four
hours suggests a pathological cause of the cyanosis.

Cyanosis without dyspnea usually occurs with hypoglycemia or if the baby is chilled. Cyanosis due to congenital heart lesions with respiratory distress in the
first few days of life requires emergency workup. These
findings are present in infants with pulmonary atresia
with intact ventricular septum, pulmonary atresia with
ventricular septal defect, malformation of the tricuspid
valve, tricuspid atresia, transposition of the great arteries, total anomalous pulmonary venous return, hypo-
plastic left heart, and some with coarctation of the aorta.

Pallor in a newborn, in contrast to the older child,
is due almost always to circulatory failure, anoxia, edema
or shock. Only rarely will a severe neonatal anemia without shock be manifested by pallor. An infant who remains
pallid may have respiratory obstruction, cerebral anoxia,
narcosis, cerebral hemorrhage, hypoglycemia, cretinism
or circulatory failure due to adrenal hemorrhage. The
pallor of anoxia is usually associated with bradycardia,

and the pallor of anemia with tachycardia. Postmature
infants tend to have pallid skins. A beefy red color of the
skin may also indicate hypoglycemia in an infant born to
a diabetic mother or may indicate poorly developed vasomotor reflexes. Occasionally, one half of the body may
appear red and the other half pale: the harlequin color
change of the newborn. This usually is transient and of
unknown significance. Plethora may also occur from
twin-twin transfusion, maternal-fetal transfusion and in
the adrenogenital syndrome. Alternating pink and blue
patches may be due to transient vessel abnormalities or
to cutis marmorata.

Injuries secondary to delivery or application of for-
ceps are recorded. Scratches, petechiae and ecchymoses
are most frequently due to injuries incident to delivery.
However, petechiae and ecchymoses in the newborn are
also caused by sepsis, erythroblastosis fetalis, hemorrhagic disease of the newborn and thrombocytopenic purpura. Rarely, purpuric spots are due to hemophilia and
diseases such as toxoplasmosis, syphilis or cytomegalic
inclusion disease and may occur in infants whose mothers
had rubella during the first trimester.

Any tumors or hemangiomas are noted. Telangiec-
tases or capillary hemangiomas are frequently found at
the back of the neck, the base of the nose, the center of
the forehead and on the eyelids, nevus flammeus. Vascular nevi may appear elsewhere. Pigmented nevi are the
common birthmarks and may appear any time during the
first year of life. Size, shape, color and degree of protuberance should be recorded.

The skin of the newborn normally feels puffy and
edematous. Excess edema may be noted in premature infants, in infants born of diabetic or prediabetic mothers or
edematous mothers, or in infants with hydrops due to
blood -- especially Rh -- incompatibility. It is rarely
noted in children with abnormal salt retention or hypo-
proteinemia.

Localized edema may be noted in a presenting hand
or foot or other presenting part due to trauma. Edema
limited to the hands and feet may be a sign of neonatal
tetany. Edema of the genitals in both sexes is common

especially in those infants born by breech delivery. Edema of the anterior abdominal wall suggests perforation of a viscus with peritonitis, or obstructive uropathy.

Poor turgor and excessive wrinkling may indicate dehydration. Dehydration of the infant immediately after birth may indicate poor maternal nutrition, maternal toxemia, defective placenta, or sepsis of the newborn. Large babies with good turgor may be born of mothers with diabetes or may occur in cretins.

The vernix caseosa, a cheesy white material, is found in the skin folds and the nail beds. Yellow discoloration of the vernix occurs with intrauterine distress, post-maturity, hemolytic disease of the newborn and, occasionally, in infants born by breech presentation.

Desquamation occurs normally in all infants and may be generalized. Marked peeling and cracking of the skin occurs in dysmature infants. Small hard scales may indicate congenital ichthyosis (collodion babies).

Redness of the skin with red pinpoint macules and papules developing in the first days of life are usually transitory rashes caused by irritation, toxicity or unknown cause. Erythema toxicum may appear within the first three days of life and may be indistinguishable from miliaria, heat rash or varicella. Erythema toxicum has a red base; miliaria does not.

Pustules should be examined carefully. Pinpoint white spots, usually over the bridge of the nose, chin or cheeks, are most frequently milia due to retained sebum and are not true pustules. Small pustules following water-drop-like miliaria are a form of miliaria, miliaria crystallina or miliaria pustulosa. Small pustules with surrounding red areas are diagnostic of impetigo neonatorum. If these pustules are associated with bullae, pemphigus is present. Pemphigus of the palms and soles of the newborn suggests congenital syphilis. Tender, red, indurated areas with sharp borders, due to streptococcal infection, are termed erysipelas. In the newborn, erysipelas may be found near the umbilicus or at the site of a skin injury. Vesiculobullous lesions in the newborn may also be due to infection by viruses of herpes simplex, varicella, or

variola-vaccinia if the mother is infected at the time of
delivery.

Small discrete bullous patches involving the deeper
layers of the skin, usually with large hemorrhagic areas,
are called "epidermolysis bullosa." Small reddish or
purple areas of the skin which are hard and movable, fat
necrosis, may be due to trauma during or after delivery
but may indicate hypercalcemia. These areas with hard
edges feel like small saucers or like small loose peas
under the skin.

Redness, starting on the face and extending over the
entire body and appearing in the second week of life, associated with desquamation of large patches of skin, is
diagnostic of dermatitis exfoliativa (Ritter's disease). In
this condition, large patches of epithelium can be removed
by stroking the skin (Nikolsky's sign). Redness and desquamation in the skin folds represent intertrigo, usually
caused by sweating and chafing but sometimes caused by
fungal or other infections.

It is sometimes difficult to determine the presence
of jaundice in the newborn. As in the older child, one
looks at the skin, the sclerae, the mucous membranes
and the nail beds in natural daylight. Minimal jaundice in
a plethoric newborn may be more easily obtained by placing
a glass slide on the infant's cheek. With slight pressure,
the capillary blood and erythema will fade but the yellowness caused by the jaundice will remain, making the jaundice more easily discernible. Jaundice is usually visible
in the child or adult when the serum bilirubin reaches
2 mg. per cent. It may not be visible in the newborn until
the level is 5 mg. per cent, probably because there is
less fat in the newborn subcutaneous tissue in which bilirubin is soluble. Jaundice is usually not seen at birth because light is required to develop the pigment.

Jaundice in newborns apparently progresses from
the head to the feet. Levels of serum bilirubin can be
roughly estimated from the most caudal area of the body
which is jaundiced:

Head alone   5-8 mg. per cent

Head and chest	6-12
To knees	8-16
Including arms and lower legs	10-18
Including hands and feet	15-20+

Jaundice appearing at birth or within 12 hours thereafter is almost diagnostic of erythroblastosis fetalis. Jaundice after 24 hours is usually physiological but may also
be due to erythroblastosis secondary to Rh or A-B-O incompatibility; sepsis, congenital syphilis, hemolytic icterus, bile duct obstruction or viral hepatitis. Physiologic jaundice usually disappears in the full-term infant by
the second week, but may persist without obvious cause
for as long as four weeks. Persistent "physiologic" jaundice of the newborn for longer than four weeks may be seen
in infants with congenital heart disease, especially with
heart failure, or cretinism. Sepsis with jaundice is usually due to staphylococci or Escherichia coli. Sepsis
without jaundice is usually due to streptococci or pneumococci. Lethargy may be associated with jaundice from
any cause.

Sweating is rare in the newborn, but may be present
in babies with brain cortex irritation, anomalies or injuries of the sympathetic nervous system, or in babies
whose mothers were morphine addicts.

Congenital skin anomalies and deformities are common and should be noted. A soft swelling, especially of
the tongue or over the clavicle, which contains fluid and
transilluminates, is usually a lymphangioma or cystic
hygroma. Midline cysts of the neck may be thyroglossal
cysts. Small holes or defects anywhere in the neck, and
extending up to the ear, may be branchial clefts or cysts.

Bluish pigmentation over the sacrum, buttocks, or
back or occasionally over the extensor surfaces, is termed
Mongolian spots. They are due to pigment cells in the deep
layers of the skin, usually disappear in later life when the
superficial pigment masks them, and have no clinical significance.

Examine all skin folds to be certain that the skin
moves over the underlying bone. Constricting bands,

which are associated with deformity or atrophy beyond the contracture, may be hidden by the folds in the obese infant.

Ectodermal defects of the scalp are common. These usually appear as large firm sharply demarcated patches without hair. Look for small holes in the midline of the scalp or anywhere along the spinal column which may be dermal sinuses and, if infected, may be a cause of recurrent meningitis. A defect along this same area with hair over the defect is usually a spina bifida. If neural structures protrude through the defect, the mass is termed an "encephalocele" if on the head or a "meningomyelocele" if over the spine.

Generalized hardness of the skin is termed "sclerema." This condition may be due to over-cooling of the infant and is prone to occur in debilitated infants, particularly if they have marked alterations in their serum electrolytes. Patchy areas of induration of the skin -- hidebound skin -- is scleroderma and usually does not occur in the newborn.

NAILS

The nail beds should be pink. Yellowing of the nail beds has the same significance as yellowing of the vernix. Melanin is normally found in the newborn Negro in the nail beds and near the genitalia in increased amounts. Absence or defects of the nails are usually congenital and may represent a form of ectodermal dysplasia. The nails may be short in premature infants and unusually long in postmature infants.

Other diseases are described in the general discussion of the skin.

TONE

Usually at birth the infant is limp, but after the first or second cry he develops good muscle tone. Shortly after birth, the newborn infant flexes himself in a "position of comfort," the position he occupied in utero. Areas of flaccidity or spasticity are noted.

Poor muscle tone in an infant a few minutes of age should be regarded as a grave sign. Infants who remain limp longer than a few minutes should be suspected of having anoxia, narcosis, central nervous system lesions, particularly edema or hemorrhage, vascular collapse, hypoglycemia or mongolism. A few newborns with myasthenia gravis have been noted to be limp; these have been born of mothers with the disease. Many infants, however, who have been limp for longer than several hours eventually appear to be normal. Cause of prolonged limpness in these is usually not adequately explained. Local loss of muscle tone may indicate a peripheral nerve lesion. Excess muscle tone may indicate central nervous system or metabolic muscular disease.

Convulsions rarely are present at birth. They may be distinguished from normal tremulousness in that the convulsing child is usually quiet before the seizure; the tremulous child is usually active. Shortly after birth, convulsions indicate anoxia, increased intracranial pressure due to bleeding or infection, anomalies of the central nervous system, or hypocalcemia with tetany. Rarely, omphalitis due to Clostridium tetani causes tetanus of the newborn with convulsions. Infants with hypoglycemia may have convulsions, and very rarely neonatal nephritis causes convulsions. Muscular twitching and hypertonicity are similar in diagnostic significance as convulsions. However, tremors and twitchings of short duration may be noted, especially if the infant is cold or startled; these are usually normal and occur in active infants. In infants, overalertness with twitching may result from narcotic withdrawal if the mother is addicted, or rarely may indicate hyperthyroidism. Asymmetrical seizures do not help distinguish metabolic from intracranial causes. Seizures due to hypocalcemia or infection usually begin after the fourth day of life; those due to anoxia, birth injury, anomalies, or hypoglycemia in the first three days.

A few facies are characteristic at this age. Mongolian facies can usually be recognized at birth, but cretinism is usually not detectable until about six weeks of age. Gargoylism can be detected if suspected, but is usually not diagnosed for several months. The facies of

a newborn with renal agenesis is characterized by low
ears, senile appearance, broad nose and receding chin.
Multiple fractures are noted in children with osteogenesis
imperfecta. Disproportion of one side of the body indicates
absence or abnormalities of the bones or muscles, or congenital hypertrophy. Other facies are described in
Chapter III.

HEAD

Especially one notes the presence and amount of over-
riding of sutures. Immediately after birth the fontanels
may appear to be very small or entirely closed, and the
suture lines will be represented by hard ridges. These
findings are normal and are considered part of the molding process of a normal vaginal delivery. Within the first
day of life, the normal intracranial pressure begins to ex-
ert its expansive force, and the suture lines and fontanels
are felt as depressions in the normal infant. The progress
of this expansion is followed during the entire period of infancy but especially during the neonatal period. Failure
of normal expansion in the neonatal period may be the
earliest sign of microcephaly or craniostenosis. Contrari-
wise, rapid enlargement of the fontanels is not a good early
sign of developing hydrocephalus: absolute measurements
of skull and chest circumference are necessary for this
diagnosis. Anencephaly and congenital hydrocephaly are
obvious at birth.

A tense fontanel any time after birth and until the
fontanel closes indicates increased intracranial pressure.
Except in those infants whose intracranial pressure is
raised because of crying or coughing, a tense or bulging
fontanel usually indicates a disease of pediatric emergency
status, as already discussed. A depressed fontanel may
be normal or may be an early indication of dehydration in
the newborn infant. A third fontanel, located between the
anterior and posterior fontanels, may be a sign of mongolism or other form of "at-risk" infant.

Cephalohematoma is noted; frequently the hematoma
is not present at birth but appears on the second day. The
hematoma is soft, fluctuant, and the outline well defined
with the edge at the bone margin. If the cephalohematoma

crosses the midline, fracture of the skull is present. A cephalohematoma begins to calcify in the first few days of life, and a ridge around the hematoma may be felt for as long as six months.

In contrast to the cephalohematoma, the caput succedaneum is soft but ill defined in outline, pits on pressure and is not fluctuant. This represents only edema of the scalp, perhaps due to pressure on the emissary veins. The presence of caput should be noted as this may indicate difficult delivery with possible intracranial hemorrhage.

The examiner presses the scalp behind and above the ears with the fingers, as if playing the piano, to determine the presence of a ping-pong ball sensation, craniotabes. Many normal newborns have craniotabes, but if it is present, hydrocephalus and syphilis should also be suspected. The other causes of craniotabes, which have been discussed, occur later in life.

Cranial or facial asymmetry is common and is usually due to intrauterine molding or to molding during delivery. Facial or cranial asymmetry may occur in infants with facial palsy, but usually infants with facial nerve injury are not born with asymmetry. Facial asymmetry may occur in infants of low birth weight and associated hemihypertrophy (Silver's syndrome). Micrognathia, small jaw, if present may be a cause of cyanosis.

Head retraction may be a sign of a vascular ring causing respiratory obstruction.

Chvostek's sign is usually positive in the normal newborn infant and therefore of little value in diagnosing neonatal tetany.

EYES

If the infant is crying or keeps his eyes shut, gently rock his head. Usually he will open his eyes by this maneuver long enough for a thorough examination.

The presence and structure of the eyes are noted. Real tears may not appear until the second month and the lacrimal ducts may not open until several weeks later. Purulent discharge from the eyes shortly after birth usually signifies ophthalmia neonatorum due to gonorrhea.

While any discharge from the eyes may begin on the first day of life, usually chemical irritation causes discharge on days 1-3, gonorrhea between days 2-5, and inclusion blennorrhea due to viral infection on days 4-14.

A mongoloid slant, the lateral upward slope of the eyes with an inner epicanthal fold, or an antimongoloid slant may be noted. While these may be variants of the normal, they may suggest one of the major syndromes of mental, physical or chromosomal aberrations.

Exophthalmos at this age is usually a congenital anomaly with enlargement of all the structures of the eye -- buphthalmos. However, congenital glaucoma occurs and is a cause of exophthalmos in the newborn. An open-eyed stare, common in newborn infants with cerebral palsy, may be confused with exophthalmos.

Enophthalmos is usually associated with ptosis and constricted pupil, Horner's syndrome, and at this age indicates damage to the brain or to the cervical spine and brachial plexus root. Constricted pupil alone, unilateral dilated fixed pupil, nystagmus or strabismus may be an early sign of brain injury. A searching nystagmus is not uncommon at birth. Later, this type of nystagmus may indicate blindness. An intermittent strabismus is present in nearly all infants at birth, but disappears by six months.

Conjunctival or scleral hemorrhages are common and usually have no clinical significance. They may, however, indicate difficult delivery or hemorrhagic disease of the newborn. Conjunctival edema and discharge may appear a few days after birth and are usually due to chemicals or eye infections.

The cornea is examined. Anomalies of the cornea and pupil are noted. Keratitis at this age may be due to trauma but usually signifies gonorrhea. The corneal reflex should be present at birth, but is tested only if brain or eye damage is suspected. Haziness may indicate cataract or glaucoma. Congenital cataracts may indicate maternal rubella, galactosemia or disorders of calcium metabolism.

The retina is examined and a red reflex is obtained. If the infant keeps his eyes closed, raising his head with one hand is often helpful in getting him to open them long enough to visualize the retina. Absence of the red reflex,

if the examination is performed properly, may indicate the
presence of lens opacities or retinoblastoma. Retinal hemorrhages usually indicate subdural hematoma or other brain
trauma. Choreoretinitis due to congenital toxoplasmosis
or cytomegalic inclusion disease may be found.

The pupil of the newborn may be constricted for about
three weeks, or may respond to light at birth by contracting,
the pupillary reflex. Absence of the reflex after three weeks
suggests that the infant is blind or may have suffered intracranial anoxia or oculomotor nerve damage.

EARS

Anomalies, position, and injuries of the external
ear are noted. Low-set ears may be associated with renal
agenesis or chromosomal abnormalities. The canals are
usually filled with vernix and amniotic debris, so that the
drums may not be visualized at birth. Usually, the drums
are easily visualized at a few days of age. Branchial
clefts are noted. Deafness can be determined at a few
days of age by snapping the fingers or making a sharp
noise. Normally, the eyelids will twitch or a complete
Moro reflex will be obtained. In the newborn with deafness, there is no such response. Congenital deafness,
filled aural canals, congenital syphilis or kernicterus
should be suspected.

NOSE

The nose is usually deformed for a few days after
birth, but injury is rare. Patency of the nasal canals may
be tested by holding the hand over the baby's mouth and
noting the normal passage of air. Mucus is usually present in the nose of the newborn. A more certain method of
testing nasal patency is to pass a soft rubber catheter with
suction, as already described. Non-patent nasal airway at
this age is usually due to choanal atresia or other congenital anomaly. Occasionally a tumor or encephalocele may
be seen protruding. Nasal discharge may be present normally, and sneezing is common. Thick bloody nasal dis-

charge without sneezing suggests congenital syphilis
(snuffles). Sneezing may occur in infants whose mothers
were receiving reserpine or narcotics and in cretins.

MOUTH

Hare-lip and cleft palate are noted.

The mouth is always opened to search for anomalies.
Because of the normally high-arched palate, it may be difficult to visualize the mouth beyond the uvula. Ordinarily,
it is not necessary to visualize beyond this point. A large
tongue usually is due to tumor (lymphangioma or hemangioma). A protruding adderlike tongue is seen with brain injury. The frenulum of the tongue may be prominent, but
usually does not restrict motion of the tongue. The sucking
reflex obtained by placing the tongue blade on the lips and
noting the child suck, and the rooting reflex, obtained by
touching the cheek and noting the infant turn and suck, are
normal reflexes present at birth. Absence of these reflexes occurs in brain-injured or debilitated infants, and
in some normal infants for the first day or two of life.

Teeth may be present at birth. Retention cysts or
pearls are common along the gum margins. Flat white
spots which do not rub away -- thrush -- may be present
by three or four days of life. Small hard tumors may be
seen in the gingiva, especially in the incisor area (epulis).
Ulcers or plaques may be seen on the hard palate, usually
due to vigorous sucking, after a few days of age (Bednar's
aphthae). Small white epithelial cysts along both sides of
the median raphe of the hard palate are Epstein's pearls.

Tonsillar tissue is not seen in the newborn.

Vomiting is a symptom in older children but may be
considered a sign in the newborn. It is common in the infant of one or two days of age and may be due only to relaxation of the cardia of the stomach. It has such various
causes as cerebral anoxia, increased intracranial pressure, sepsis, marked jaundice, adrenal hyperplasia, peritonitis; and intestinal obstruction due to volvulus, tracheoesophageal fistula, malrotation, annular pancreas, diaphragmatic hernia, atresia of the intestine, meconium

ileus, bands, diverticuli, duplications, imperforate anus, Hirschsprung's disease or cretinism.

Vomiting of uncurdled milk or prompt vomiting of anything occurs in infants with esophageal atresia, but it also occurs in normal infants who have been fed too much or too fast or who have not been properly "burped" or positioned after feeding. Passage of a catheter with suction, as described, helps to determine presence of esophageal atresia. Bloody vomitus in the newborn most commonly is due to ingested blood, but occasionally occurs with hemorrhagic disease of the newborn or with gastrointestinal ulcers associated with intracranial anoxia or increased pressure. Vomitus with bile suggests an obstruction below the ampulla of Vater or perforation of a viscus; without bile, obstruction above the ampulla. Fecal vomiting usually indicates a low intestinal obstruction. Vomiting also occurs in children with electrolyte disturbances, urinary tract disease or infections.

Saliva is usually scant until the second or third month of life. Profuse salivation with mucoid secretions in the newborn may indicate the presence of tracheoesophageal fistula or cystic fibrosis, but may frequently be due to tracheal aspiration or tracheal irritation.

NECK

In the supine position the newborn's neck is generally not visible. Bring the neck into full vision by placing one hand behind the upper back and allow the head to fall gently into extension.

Distended neck veins usually signify a mass in the chest or pneumomediastinum. A mass in the lower part of the sternocleidomastoid muscle with limitation of motion of the neck results in torticollis. Small cystic masses in the region of the upper part of the sternocleidomastoid may be branchial cleft cysts. A fractured clavicle may present as a mass in the neck. A midline mass may be a congenital goiter, which is rare, or a thyroglossal duct cyst, which is more common. A soft mass over the clavicle which transilluminates may be a cystic hygroma.

An unusually short neck which is poorly mobile may be an indication of the Klippel-Feil syndrome; skin folds from the acromion to the mastoid may indicate gonadal dysgenesis. Excess posterior cervical skin may indicate other chromosomal aberration.

The neck is flexed. **Resistance** is rare but may indicate meningeal irritation. To the contrary, however, lack of resistance does not indicate lack of meningeal irritation, as a newborn infant with meningitis may have a supple neck.

The neck is turned from side to side to obtain the tonic neck reflex which is normally present in the newborn. Absence of this reflex may indicate central nervous system damage. When the head is turned with the infant supine, the trunk should rotate in the direction of the head movement, the neck-righting reflex. Similarly, if the body is tilted in the erect infant, the head should return to the upright position, a labyrinth response (otolith-righting reflex).

The cry of the infant is noted. The infant should cry lustily at birth. A weak or groaning cry or grunt in expiration usually indicates severe respiratory disturbances. Absence or weakness of cry or constant crying at birth usually indicates brain injury. A high-pitched (or cerebral) cry may indicate increased intracranial pressure. Hoarseness or crowing inspirations may indicate laryngeal disease or anomalies: laryngeal or thyroglossal tumor, congenital laryngeal stridor, laryngeal paralysis, stenosis of the larynx or trachea, congenital heart disease, vascular ring, tracheomalacia, tracheal webs or other causes extrinsic to the larynx. Hoarseness appearing at two to five days of age frequently is due to laryngospasm caused by hypocalcemia. Hoarseness is usually absent in congenital laryngeal stridor; therefore, its presence requires study.

CHEST

The chest is examined for gross anomalies, tumors or fractures. The chest is usually almost circular in the newborn. Depressed sternum may be due to atelectasis, respiratory distress syndrome or funnel chest. The xiphisternum protrudes and appears broken, normally. This is due to weak attachment of the xiphoid with the body of the sternum. Retractions usually indicate interference with air entry. Marked retraction of the chest suggests upper airway, particularly laryngeal, obstruction such as laryngeal stenosis. Immediate direct laryngoscopy is indicated.

Asymmetry of the chest may be due to diaphragmatic hernia or paralysis, pneumothorax, emphysema, tension cysts, pleural effusions, pneumonia or pulmonary agenesis. An asymmetrical mass near the neck may be a fractured clavicle. Palpation may reveal congenital absence of a clavicle or of muscle.

Enlargement of the breasts due to maternal hormones usually is seen on the second or third day in either sex and may persist normally as long as a month. Milky secretions may be present. Redness and firmness around the nipple is rare and is due to infection -- mastitis or abscess. Increased pigmentation of the areola is found in the adrenogenital syndrome.

LUNGS

The newborn infant's respiration is chiefly abdominal. Decreased abdominal respiration is noted in infants with pulmonary disease or distended abdomen. Thoracic breathing or unequal motion of the chest is noted in infants with phrenic nerve paralysis, diaphragmatic hernia or massive atelectasis. Unequal motion of the chest or deep retraction of the sternum, especially if associated with rapid, gasping, or grunting respiration or flaring nares, is most important in indicating intrathoracic disease.

Respiratory rate is 30 to 50 at birth. Respiratory movements are irregular in rate and depth in the normal newborn. Weak, irregular, slow or very rapid rates suggest brain damage. Grunting rapid respirations may be the only sign of a very sick infant, and may be due to

overwhelming infections anywhere in the body, lung, heart
or brain diseases, anemia or distended abdomen.

Deep sighing respirations are noted frequently in
infants with acidosis. Cheyne-Stokes type of respiration
or weak, groaning respiration may be a sign of hypoxia
or brain damage in the full-term infant.

The cough reflex is usually absent in the newborn
but appears in a day or two.

In percussing or auscultating the chest one must
observe that the child lies so that the head and neck are
not turned. Increased or decreased areas of dullness
or changes in breath sounds may occur simply because
of the position of the infant.

The chest is resonant shortly after birth. Hyperresonance suggests emphysema but is more often due to
pneumomediastinum, pneumothorax or diaphragmatic
hernia. Decreased resonance indicates improper aeration, usually due to atelectasis, occasionally to pneumonia, respiratory distress syndrome or empyema. Atelectasis may represent primary failure of expansion of the
lung, or may be due to aspiration of amniotic fluid, food
or other foreign body, thyroid or possibly thymic tumors,
other mediastinal masses, diaphragmatic hernia or
chylothorax.

Auscultation should reveal bronchial breath sounds
bilaterally. Air entry should be good, particularly in the
midaxillary line. An expiratory grunt suggests difficult
air exchange. Rales usually indicate normal newborn
atelectasis. Pleuropericardial rubs have no clinical significance. Peristaltic sounds may be heard in the chest
with diaphragmatic hernia, though these sounds are frequently transmitted from the abdomen in normal infants.
If breath sounds are heard on both sides of the chest and
the heart sounds are heard in the usual place, diaphragmatic hernia or pneumothorax is unlikely. Intrinsic lung
diseases may cause changes in breath sounds.

A Downes score to estimate degree of respiratory
distress in infants with no pneumothorax, pneumomediastinum, or aspiration, can be obtained.

	Score		
	0	1	2
Respiratory rate	<60	61-80	>80 or apneic
Cyanosis	0	in air	in 40% O_2
Retractions	0	mild	moderate-severe
Grunt	0	with stethoscope	without stethoscope
Air entry (crying, axilla)	clear	delayed	barely audible

Such a score is useful in indicating oxygen require-
ments of the baby. A score of 0-3 represents mild distress, 4-6 moderate, and 7-10 severe.

HEART

The heart size is percussed or the apical impulse
palpated. The apex will usually be found lateral to the
midclavicular line and in the third or fourth interspace
because of the more horizontal position of the newborn
infant's heart. Dextrocardia should be noted. A large
heart at birth is found rarely with valvular heart disease, but is seen in infants born of diabetic mothers,
in infants with erythroblastosis fetalis, von Gierke's
disease, or rhabdomyoma of the heart. A few days after birth, however, cardiac enlargement may be due to
heart failure secondary to heart anomalies (e.g., coarctation of the aorta, septal defects, patent ductus arteriosus, hypoplasia of the left heart, truncus arteriosus,
anomalous coronary arteries), or to endocardial fibro-
elastosis, paroxysmal tachycardia, hypertension of any
cause or toxic myocarditis. Enlarged heart with other
signs of heart failure also may be due to peripheral
arteriovenous connections, such as cerebral arteriovenous aneurysms.

The heart rate at birth varies from 100 to 180, and
stabilizes shortly after birth at 120 to 140. The rhythm

is usually regular. Varying rhythm is associated with
anoxia, cerebral defects or increased intracranial pressure.

Murmurs are noted for loudness, quality, location
and timing, but their significance cannot usually be determined at this age. Murmurs, if present, are usually
heard at the left sternal border in the 3rd or 4th interspace, or over the base of the heart -- almost never at
the apex. Heart sounds are heard poorly with pneumothorax or pneumomediastinum, cardiac failure or central
nervous system injury. Clicking or crackling sounds
synchronous with the heart beat suggest mediastinal
emphysema.

ABDOMEN

The abdomen is usually prominent. The veins over
the abdomen are prominent normally, but are distended
in infants with peritonitis and pylephlebitis.

Visible peristaltic waves indicate intestinal obstruction but may be seen in thin, otherwise normal infants.
Peristalsis is normally heard shortly after birth. A silent
tympanitic distended tender abdomen suggests peritonitis.

Scaphoid abdomen may be noted in children with diaphragmatic hernia or high atresia of the intestinal tract.
The abdomen may be distended with ascites, low intestinal
obstruction such as atresia of the ileum or colon, imperforate anus or meconium plug; peritonitis or ileus,
tracheoesophageal fistula, omphalocele, enlargement
of abdominal organs or Hirschsprung's disease.

Ascites may be due to any of the causes listed under
edema and, in addition, may be due to ruptured viscus,
chylous ascites, peritonitis, necrotizing enterocolitis,
hepatitis, cirrhosis, congenital anomalies causing obstruction of the portal vein or to urethral obstruction or other
genitourinary anomalies.

The liver is normally palpated 2-3 cm. below the
right costal margin. The spleen tip is usually palpable at
about one week of age. Enlarged liver and spleen are usually palpated or percussed in infants with erythroblastosis
fetalis, sepsis, trauma to liver or spleen, or congenital

syphilis. Enlarged liver and spleen are found also in infants born of diabetic mothers, and perhaps in infants
with congenital hemolytic icterus.

Left-sided liver is usually associated with situs inversus. Other malrotations are usually not detected by
physical examination.

The lower one-half of the right and tip of the left
kidney are normally palpated. One cannot diagnose agenesis of the kidney, however, simply if the kidney is not felt.
If the infant is crying, palpation for the kidneys may be
facilitated by supporting the infant at a 45-degree angle
with one hand at the occiput and neck. Palpate the abdomen
with the free hand, and simultaneously flex the neck with
the other hand. Abdominal muscles will relax, and the
infant usually stops crying. Flexing the knees to the
abdomen sometimes also gives enough relaxation. Enlarged kidneys may be noted with neuroblastoma, Wilms's
tumor, polycystic kidneys or congenital hydronephrosis. A
single enlarged kidney may indicate renal vein thrombosis.

The bladder is normally percussed or palpated 1-4
cm. above the symphysis. Ironically, a greatly distended
bladder is palpated with great difficulty in the newborn because of its very thin wall, and it must be percussed or it
will be overlooked. Distended bladder may be due to congenital bladder-neck or urethral obstruction.

Any other masses palpable in the abdomen must be
identified. Tumors, meconium ileus, loculated hemorrhage or other abnormal masses may be found.

The umbilical cord is inspected. If the amnion cov-
ers the umbilical stump, the condition is called "amniotic
navel"; if covered by skin,"cutis navel." Neither has any
clinical significance except that the first may be associated with delayed healing and the second may be mistaken
for umbilical hernia. A velamentous cord with insertion
near the edge is rare but may signify other anomalies.
The umbilical cord normally has two arteries and should
be examined for this. One artery may be accompanied by
other anomalies.

The cord should be noted to be dry and not bleeding.
If bleeding, the cord must be re-tied. Redness around the

cord after 24 hours, wetness of the stump, or a fetid odor after three days usually signifies the presence of omphalitis. A cord which fails to drop off after two weeks, or a navel which persists in draining after three weeks may indicate the presence of a urachal cyst or sinus. Similarly, a child born with a very large and flabby umbilical cord may have a patent urachus. Fecal discharge occurs with a persistent omphalomesenteric duct and this in turn usually indicates the presence of a Meckel's diverticulum. Patent omphalomesenteric duct may result in ileal prolapse, a surgical emergency.

Soft granulation tissue is commonly seen following cord separation. This is a local condition which must be distinguished from the firmer umbilical polyp, which is dark red, has a mucoid discharge and is related to Meckel's diverticulum. Other cysts and tumors of the umbilicus occur rarely.

Ventral hernias with or without diastasis recti are frequently present at birth and are usually insignificant. Very large hernias, omphalocele, may be incompatible with life. Occasionally a child is born with a hernia which pinches off the small bowel.

GENITALIA

The genitalia are inspected. Edema is common especially in children born by breech delivery. Pigmentation is usually increased around the genitalia in dark-skinned races but may be a sign of adrenal hyperplasia. Femoral pulses, hydrocele and hernia are noted. Though the clitoris is always large, careful inspection of the labiae is indicated. An unusually large clitoris is found in pseudo-hermaphroditism, usually due to adrenal hyperplasia. What appears to be a large clitoris may be a small penis. Therefore, the urethral opening should be identified. In the female, the urethral opening is just back of the clitoris. In the male, if the opening is on the ventral surface of the penis, hypospadias exists; if on the dorsal surface, epispadias. Ulceration of the urethral orifice may occur in the newborn, especially following circumcision.

A tight <u>prepuce</u> is usually found in newborn males; phimosis does not exist unless the prepuce cannot be pulled back just far enough to allow the flow of a good urinary stream. The prepuce should not be retracted more than is adequate for examination. Small bands and adhesions of the prepuce are usually broken during the examination. Erection and even priapism may be noted in the newborn, but are usually without clinical significance.

The <u>labiae</u>, especially the labiae minora, are usually large in the newborn female. The normal labiae may be confused with a bifid scrotum. Adhesions of the labiae minora may occur shortly after birth. Vaginal mucoid or bloody <u>discharge</u> may occur normally in the female due to maternal hormones, may appear any time in the first week, and may persist as long as a month. The catheter previously used may now be used again. The opening of the hymen should be visualized. Passing the catheter through the hymenal opening tests for both imperforate hymen and vaginal atresia.

The <u>testes</u>, whether in the canal or scrotum, should be palpated. The <u>scrotum</u> may appear large, especially after breech delivery. Hydroceles and herniae are noted. A unilateral dark swollen non-tender testis may be a sign of testicular infarction of the newborn.

Femoral pulses are palpated. Absence suggests coarctation of the aorta.

Fecal urethral discharges may be present. They indicate rectourethral, rectovaginal or rectovesical fistulas.

SPINE

The infant is then placed on his abdomen. The hand is run lightly over the spine. Spina bifida, pilonidal sinus, scoliosis, and the anal dimple are sought. If the <u>anus</u> does not appear patent, the previously used catheter should be inserted. If the abdomen is distended, rectal examination should be performed immediately.

MECONIUM, URINE

Though usually not considered part of the physical examination, note must be made of the passage of meconium and urine. The newborn usually voids immediately at birth or within a short time of birth. Failure to pass urine by 24 hours of age is a highly suggestive sign of urinary tract obstruction or other urinary tract anomaly and requires further investigation.

Meconium is usually passed during the first three days of life. Passage of meconium before birth is diagnostic of fetal intrauterine distress. Failure of passage of meconium by the end of the second day of life suggests an intestinal tract obstruction. Passage of small amounts of meconium, or passage of meconium over a long period of time, suggests a high intestinal or partial intestinal obstruction. Presence of bright red blood in the meconium is usually due to ingested mother's blood by the baby, but may be due to hemorrhage somewhere in the intestinal tract -- an emergency distinction which must be made by suitable laboratory tests.

EXTREMITIES

The infant is replaced on his back. Gently "fold" the infant into his intrauterine position. This will make him relax and he may even sleep. It also provides a clue to the range of motion which is normal to that child. For example, a child whose hips and knees are drawn to one side in utero will have a greater range of motion of the abducted hip than the adducted hip. Extremities are noted. Fingers are counted. Polydactyly and syndactyly are noted. Fractures, paralyses and dislocations are felt for, and the hips are examined for dislocation by rotating the thighs with the knees flexed. Soft clicks are common when hips are moved, as described in Chapter VII. These must be distinguished from the sharp click of dislocation. Clicks at the knees are also common. Multiple fractures with deformity may be due to osteogenesis imperfecta. Paralysis of the arm may be due to brachial palsy or fractured humerus. Paralysis of both legs is usually due to severe trauma or congenital anomaly of the spinal cord. The hands are normally held clenched. Elbows, hips, and knees generally lack full extension. Response to pain and touch are noted but ordinarily not recorded. Tone of the muscle groups is noted. Passive tonus is also tested by moving all the major joints. Paralysis, missed during examination of tone, may be detected. Other nerve and muscle injuries can be examined as described for the older child.

MEASUREMENTS

The head, chest, and abdominal circumferences and the length of the infant are measured and recorded. The head at birth should be 0.5 cm. or more larger than the chest or abdomen. If there is any question about developing hydrocephalus, measurements should be repeated at daily intervals.

The temperature is taken by rectum with the infant prone; in the axilla, groin or in other areas if indicated. Temperatures of 92-94 F. are common in the newborn and rise when the infant is warmed. Low temperatures are noted also after severe birth trauma and severe infection.

Elevated temperatures are noted frequently in the newborn who is dehydrated, when there is brain damage or sepsis or when the environmental temperature is excessively high. If the temperature elevation at the feet and abdomen is almost the same, the fever is usually due to the environment; if the temperature of the feet is low and that of the abdomen high, sepsis is more likely.

NEUROLOGICAL STATUS

Finally, the infant's crib is slapped or dropped a few inches and the Moro reflex, as detailed in the neurological examination, is carefully observed. This response, or the lack of it, is valuable in determining the status of the central nervous system, fractures of the arms and legs, brachial plexus injury, congenital dislocation of the

hip or recent fracture of the clavicle. An infant with
fractured clavicle may move his arm freely after 24 hours.
In infants with Erb's palsy the arm does not move due to
paralysis after brachial plexus injury. In apparent Erb's
palsy decrease in passive as well as active motion indicates an injury to the proximal humeral epiphysis. The
Moro is absent at birth and improves in infants with
cerebral edema. The Moro may be present at birth and
disappear in infants with cerebral hemorrhage.

Alternatively, the Perez reflex, another mass reflex, may be obtained. With the baby prone on a hard surface, thumb pressure is exerted from the pelvis to the
neck. A strong cry will be noted in the normal infant, together with flexion of the lower and upper extremities,
lordosis of the spine, elevation of the pelvis and head and
urination and defecation. Its significance is similar to
that of the Moro.

The infant is then re-dressed and replaced in his
crib.

Before leaving the delivery room inspect and weigh
the placenta. Amnion nodosum or vernix granuloma may
reflect insufficiency of amniotic fluid as in Potter's syndrome. Single umbilical artery is associated with certain
congenital anomalies, particularly renal, and with chromosomal trisomies.

Hydramnios, excess amniotic fluid, occurs in infants
of diabetic, pre-eclamptic or anemic mothers, in multiple
pregnancies or in infants with anencephaly, gastrointestinal
obstruction or anomalies of the great vessels.

EXAMINATION OF THE PREMATURE INFANT

A premature infant is one who at birth weighs less
than 5-1/2 lbs. (2,500 Gm.) and is less than 18 inches
(45 cm.) long.

When a premature infant is examined, the same
principles are followed as for the examination of the full-
term infant. The examination must be even more rapid,
less complete and, above all, must be done gently and
tenderly. It is more important to get the premature in-

fant in a warm isolated area, away from the doctor, than
it is to have a complete physical examination.

Measurements of the head, chest, abdomen, length
and weight, observation for gross abnormalities, and
rapid estimate of air exchange, heart rate and skin texture usually suffice for the initial examination. If a temperature measurement is desired, it should be taken in
the axilla; temperatures of premature infants approximate
that of the environment. Examination to determine the
presence of the Moro reflex may be profitably deferred
until the infant is more than a day old, and then performed
only by rapping the crib side. Transillumination of the
head, if performed, will show large areas of light transmission.

Respirations are noted after the infant is moved to
his isolated area. Normal respiration in a premature infant is irregular and Cheyne-Stokes in type. The average
rate varies from 40-80 per minute. A slow rate, rarely
a rapid rate, or a regular respiratory rate usually indicates central nervous system depression. A rapid rate
more frequently is a prime indication of infection, usually
generalized, including omphalitis, meningitis, septicemia
or pneumonia, or of atelectasis.

Because the bony thorax is soft, each inspiration is
marked by indrawing the sternum. This collapse of the
sternum normally lessens in the first 24 hours and disappears no later than the fourth or fifth day. Persistence of
the indrawing suggests the presence of persistent atelectasis. Marked atelectasis is usually present at birth, but
diminishes with each breath. Not infrequently, an infant
does well for a few minutes or few hours, and then shows
signs of respiratory distress, including marked collapse
of the chest wall, rapid respiratory rates and cyanosis.
Respiratory distress syndrome, foreign material aspiration with secondary atelectasis, pneumothorax, infection,
severe primary atelectasis, pneumomediastinum, or
localized emphysema should be suspected. The cough
reflex is usually absent in the premature infant.

Cyanosis in a premature infant usually disappears
within a few minutes at birth. Persistent cyanosis is

similar in significance to that in a full-term infant.

The texture of the <u>skin</u> should be noted. The skin of the premature infant is thin and extremely tender: it is subject to easy bruising, bleeding and infection. His skin is more subject to injury by temperature changes, which result in hardening (sclerema), than is the full-term infant.

Certain physical signs are characteristic of normal premature infants. These include a typically round head which is larger than the chest, prominent eyes, absence of eyebrows and lashes, absence of sweat, purple mottling of the skin (cutis marmorata), extensive hair (lanugo) over much of the body, and soft nails. The neck and extremities are short, the head, hands and feet are prominent, labiae minora are prominent, and the abdomen appears full. Peristalsis is normally visible through the thin abdominal wall, and this is usually not an indication of obstruction. Bloody vomitus in a premature infant may be due to intracranial hemorrhage, peptic ulcer or swallowed blood.

Though the premature infant may remain edematous for four or five days, he usually remains dehydrated longer than the full-term. As soon as the edema fluid is absorbed, the skin of the premature becomes and remains wrinkled. Jaundice appears and disappears slowly. Many prematures have umbilical hernias, and the incidence of other hernias, especially inguinal, is higher in premature than in full-term infants. A large number of premature infants have capillary hemangiomas.

The normal premature infant may seem almost motionless for the first three or four days after birth. Then he begins to cry and make vigorous movements for a few minutes at a time. Early movements usually correspond to the time of disappearance of edema and probably to the onset of hunger. The cry is usually high-pitched in the normal premature.

The degree of prematurity can sometimes be estimated by the prominence of the signs listed in the table and their comparison with those of a term newborn infant. It is important to attempt to estimate gestational age as

Signs Useful in Estimating Gestational Age

	24 wk.	28 wk.	32 wk.	34 wk.	36 wk.	37 wk.	39 wk.	41 wk.
REFLEXES								
Moro	barely present	complete						
Sucking		present	improving	strong (synch. with swallow)				
Pupillary response to light		present						
Stepping			present	minimal ----------→		fair on toes ---------→		good on heels
Crossed extension		slight withdrawal	withdrawal	withdrawal		withdrawal extension		withdrawal extension adduction
Neck righting					present ----------→			
PHYSICAL FINDINGS								
Sole creases					anterior transverse crease only	occasional creases ant. 2/3s	sole covered with creases ----→	
Scalp hair					fine and fuzzy	fine and fuzzy	coarse and silky	
Ear					pliable–no cartilage	some cartilage	stiffened by thick cartilage	
Testes and scrotum					testes in lower canal scrotum sm. few rugae	intermediate rugae	testes pendulous scrotum full extensive rugae	

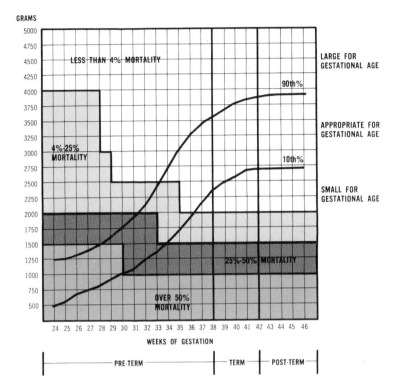

Fig. 27. Classification of newborns by birth weight, gestational age, and neonatal mortality risk. (From Battaglia, Frederick C., and Lubchenco, Lula O.: A practical classification of newborn infants by weight and gestational age, J. Pediat. 71:159-63, 1967.)

accurately as possible. Infants of low birth weight may be of decreased gestational age, or the low birth weight may be caused by various maternal, placental or fetal factors. The prognoses of these two groups differ. A classification of the newborn by birth weight, gestational age, and mortality risk is shown in Figure 27.

Because the incidence of severe congenital anomalies is higher in premature than in full-term infants,
these also must be sought, while touching the patient as
little as possible in the days immediately following his
birth.

Appendices

APPENDIX I

Record of Physical Examination

Temp._____ Pulse_____ Resp. _____ B.P. _____

Age _____ Sex _____ Ht. _____ Wt. _____

Head circ. _____ Chest circ._____

General appearance. Ill or well, distress, alert, coop-
erative, body build. Reaction to parents. Facies. Char-
acteristic position, movements, nutrition, development.
Speech.
Skin. Color, pigmentation, cyanosis. Veins, arteries,
thrombophlebitis. Jaundice, carotenemia. Pallor.
Eruptions. Petechiae. Ecchymosis. Hives. Dermato-
graphia. Tache cerebrale. Subcutaneous nodules.
Xanthomas. Texture. Scaling, striae, scars, sweat,
subcutaneous tissue, emphysema. Turgor, edema.
Nails. Cyanosis, pallor, pulsations, pitting, hemorrhages.
Hair. (Body) Distribution, color.
Lymph nodes. Occipital, post-auricular, cervical, parotid,
submaxillary, sublingual, axillary, epitrochlear, inguinal.
Size, mobility, tenderness, heat.
Head. Position, hair, shape, sutures, fontanels. Cir-
cumference. Microcephaly, hydrocephaly. Craniotabes,
Macewen's sign. Percussion, sinuses. Auscultation,
bruit, veins.
Face. Shape. Facial paralysis, trigeminal paralysis.
Swelling, parotid, submaxillary, sublingual glands. Fa-
cial appearance, hypertelorism, twitching, Chvostek's
sign.

Eyes. Vision, visual fields. Blinking. Sclerae, exophthalmos, enophthalmos. Strabismus. Ocular movement. Nystagmus. Ptosis, eyelids. Conjunctivae, pingueculae, pterygium, styes, chalazion, blepharitis. Cornea. Discharge. Pupils, accommodation, iris. Retina, red reflex, fundus, vessels, hemorrhage, chorioretinitis, disc, macula. Corneal reflex.

Ears. Anomaly, position. Discharge. Tenderness. Canals. Drums, redness, light reflex, landmarks, bulging, perforation, mobility. Mastoids, nodes. Hearing. Vestibular function.

Nose. Shape. Alae nasi, flaring. Mucosa, secretions, bleeding, airway. Septum. Polyps, tumor, encephalocele. Sinuses.

Throat. Circumoral pallor.

Lips. Paralysis, cleft, fissures, vesicles, color, edema.

Mouth. Odors, trismus. Teeth, number, edges, occlusion, caries, formation, color. Salivation.

Gums. Infection, discoloration, bleeding, cysts. Buccal mucosa, thrush, veins.

Tongue. Coating, moisture, tremor, papillae, color, geographic, furrows, scars, size, tongue-tie, cysts, paralysis.

Palate. Color, bleeding, cleft, perforation, arch. Epiglottis. Uvula, soft palate. Posterior pharynx. Tonsils, infections, size. Post-nasal drip. Koplik's, eruptions, ulcers.

Larynx. Voice. Laryngoscopy. Speech.

Neck. Size, anomalies, webbing, edema, nodes, masses. Sternocleidomastoids. Trachea. Thyroid. Vessels. Motion, opisthotonos, Brudzinski's sign, tonic neck reflex. Head drop. Tilting. Nodding.

Chest. Inspection, shape, circumference, rosary, Harrison's groove, flaring, angle, expansion; abdominal, thoracic, intercostal motion, retraction, symmetry, scapulae.

Breasts. Observation, development, symmetry, redness, heat, tenderness, masses.

Lungs. Respiration. Type, Cheyne-Stokes. Rate, tachypnea, slow, apnea, Biot. Depth, hyperpnea. Dyspnea, exercise tolerance. Cough, hemoptysis, sputum, cough reflex. Palpation, masses, tenderness, thud, fremitus; interspaces, retraction, paralysis; pulsations, friction rubs, nodes. Percussion, dullness, scapulae, diaphragm, liver, heart, mediastinum, hyperresonance. Auscultation, sounds, rales, rub, slap, rhonchi, wheezes, vocal resonance, peristalsis.

Heart. Inspection, bulging, impulse; distress, cyanosis, edema, clubbing, pulsations, vessels, femoral pulse, blood pressure. Pulse rate, tachycardia, pulsus alternans, bradycardia, water-hammer, thready, dicrotic, pulsus paradoxus. Arrhythmia, premature beats, extrasystoles, rhythm, fibrillation. Palpation, size, apex impulse, tenderness, thrill. Percussion. Auscultation, sounds, quality, split, third sound, gallop, tic-tac, friction rub, venous hum, murmurs. Failure.

Abdomen. Inspection, shape, distention, transillumination, respiration. Umbilicus, diastasis, veins. Peristalsis. Gastric waves. Auscultation. Percussion, fluid, masses. Palpation: superficial, tense, tenderness, rebound; spleen, liver, masses. Deep palpation: ballottement, bladder, kidneys, reflexes. Femoral pulses, hydration, consistency.

Genitalia. Discharge, foreign body, caruncle, prolapse. Labiae, adhesions, vagina, clitoris. Penis, hypospadias, epispadias, phimosis. Scrotum, testes, hydrocele, hernia. Cremasteric reflex, nodes.

Anus and rectum. Buttocks. Fistula. Fissure. Prolapse. Polyps. Hemorrhoids. Diaper rash. Rectum, fistula, megacolon, masses, prostate, uterus, tenderness. Sensation.

Extremities. Anomalies, length, clubbing, pain, tenderness, temperature, gangrene, swelling, deformities, shape. Feet. Gait, stance, balance, limp, ataxia.

Spine. Hair, dimples, masses, spina bifida, tenderness, mobility. Opisthotonos, scapulae. Posture, lordosis, kyphosis, scoliosis.

Joints. Heat, tenderness, swelling, effusion, redness, motion. Hips.

<u>Muscles</u>. Development, tone, tenderness, spasm, paralysis, rigidity, contractures, atrophy.
<u>Nervous system</u>. General impression, abilities, responsiveness, position, spontaneous movements, play activity, development. State of consciousness, irritability, convulsive states. Gait, stance, limp, ataxia. Coordination. Tremors, twitching, choreiform movement, athetosis, associated movements. Rigidity, paresis, paralysis, spasticity, flaccidity. Reflexes, superficial, tendon, clonus. Moro, tonic neck. Babinski, Oppenheim, Hoffmann, Kernig, Romberg, Foerster, Trousseau, peroneal, Chvostek, grasp. Thumb position. Neck and spine mobility, fontanels. Sensation, blind, deaf, withdrawal reflex, hyperesthesia, hypesthesia, position, vibration, temperature, touch. Astereognosis. Cranial nerves, I-XII. Respiratory center, circulatory center.

APPENDIX II

Denver Developmental Screening Test

(See test preceding back cover.)

The Denver Developmental Screening Test (DDST), a device for detecting developmental delays in infancy and the preschool years, has been standardized on a large cross-section of the Denver child population. The test is administered with ease and speed and lends itself to serial evaluations on the same test sheet.

<u>Test Materials.</u> Skein of red wool; box of raisins; rattle with a narrow handle; small bottle with a 5/8 inch opening; bell; tennis ball; test form; pencil; 8 one-inch cubical colored counting blocks.

<u>General Administration Instructions</u>. The mother should be told that this is a developmental screening device to obtain an estimate of the child's level of development and that it is not expected that the child be able to perform each of the test items. This test relies on observations of what the child can do and on report by a parent who

knows the child. Direct observation should be used whenever possible. Since the test requires active participation by the child, every effort should be made to put the child at ease. The younger child may be tested while sitting on the mother's lap. This should be done in such a way that he can comfortably reach the test materials on the table. The test should be administered before any frightening or painful procedures. A child will often withdraw if the examiner rushes demands upon the child. One may start by laying out one or two test materials in front of the child while asking the mother whether he performs some of the personal-social items. It is best to administer the first few test items well below the child's age level in order to assure him an initial successful experience. To avoid distractions it is best to remove all test materials from the table except the one that is being administered.

Steps in Administering the Test.

1. Draw a vertical line on the examination sheet through the four sectors (Gross Motor, Fine Motor-Adaptive, Language and Personal-Social) to represent the child's chronological age. Place the date of the examination at the top of the age line. For premature children, subtract the months of prematurity from the chronological age.

2. The items to be administered are those through which the child's chronological age line passes unless there are obvious deviations. In each sector one should establish the area where the child passes all of the items and the point at which he fails all of the items.

3. In the event that a child refuses to do some of the items requested by the examiner, it is suggested that the parent administer the item, provided she does so in the prescribed manner.

4. If a child passes an item, a large letter "P" is written on the bar at the 50 per cent passing point. "F" designates a failure, and "R" designates a refusal.

5. Note how the child adjusted to the examination, that is, his cooperation, attention span, self-confidence, and how he related to his mother, the examiner, and the test materials.

6. Ask the parent if the child's performance was typical of his performance at other times.

7. To retest the child on the same form, use a different color pencil for the scoring and age line.

8. Instructions for administering footnoted items are on the back of the test form.

Interpretations. The test items are placed into four categories: Gross Motor; Fine Motor-Adaptive; Language; and Personal-Social. Each of the test items is designated by a bar which is so located under the age scale as to indicate clearly the ages at which 25 per cent, 50 per cent, 75 per cent and 90 per cent of the standardization population could perform the particular test item. The left end of the bar designates the age at which 25 per cent of the standardization population could perform the item; the hatch mark at the top of the bar, 50 per cent; the left end of the shaded area, 75 per cent; and the right end of the bar, the age at which 90 per cent of the standardization population could perform the item.

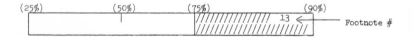

Failure to perform an item passed by 90 per cent of children of the same age should be considered significant. Such a failure may be emphasized by coloring the right end of the bar of the failed item. Several failures in one sector are considered to be abnormal. These delays may be due to:

1. The unwillingness of the child to use his ability
    a) due to temporary phenomena, such as fatigue, illness, hospitalization, separation from the parent, fear, etc.
    b) general unwillingness to do most things that are asked of him - such a condition may be just as detrimental as an inability to perform

2. An inability to perform the item due to
    a) general retardation

b) pathological factors such as deafness or neurological impairment
c) familial pattern of slow development in one or
more areas

If unexplained developmental delays are noted and are a
valid reflection of a child's abilities, he should be re-
screened a month later. If the delays persist he should
be further evaluated with more detailed diagnostic studies.

CAUTION: The DDST is not an intelligence test. It is in-
tended as a screening instrument for use in clinical practice to note whether the development of a particular child
is within the normal range.

Reprinted with the permission of William K.
Frankenburg, M. D. , and Josiah B. Dodds, Ph. D. ,
University of Colorado Medical Center.

APPENDIX III

The charts of head circumference in boys and girls
from the ages of one month to 18 years are from Gerhard
Nellhaus (Pediatrics 41:106-14, 1968). (charts on page 218)

As indicated on pp. 13-15, height and weight as well
as head circumference are important as individual measurements, but even more as a continuous record of the
growth rate of the child. At each visit these measurements should be recorded.
The charts which follow indicate the 3, 10, 25, 50,
75, 90, and 97 percentiles of one population. If a child
has been maintaining a given percentile and suddenly
deviates, illness, starvation, or overeating should be
sought. Disproportions in height and weight may be
more easily noted by comparing with the charts, but
small disproportions are almost never significant.
The percentiles on these charts are based upon repeated measurements of infants under comprehensive

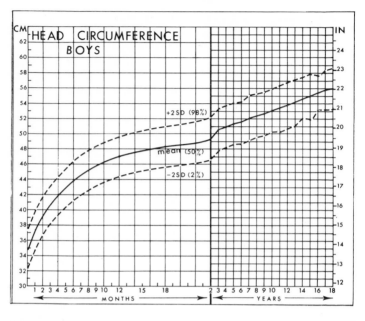

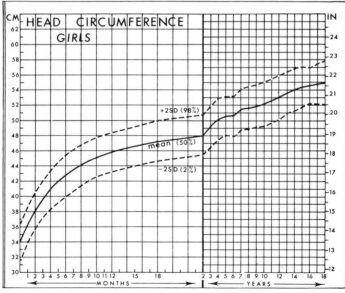

studies of health and development by Harold C. Stuart, M. D. , and associates, Department of Maternal and Child Health, Harvard School of Public Health, Boston, Massachusetts. These charts were constructed by the staff of the Department for use at the Children's Medical Center, Boston, and are reproduced with the permission of the Department and the Center.

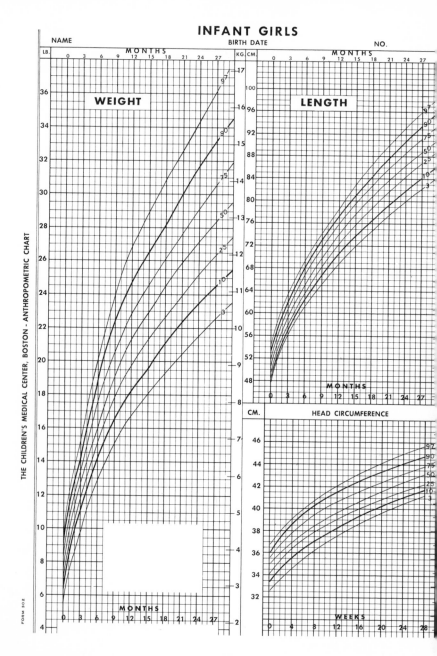

INFANT GIRLS

NAME   BIRTH DATE   NO.

WEIGHT

LENGTH

THE CHILDREN'S MEDICAL CENTER, BOSTON - ANTHROPOMETRIC CHART

HEAD CIRCUMFERENCE

MONTHS

WEEKS

FORM 302

220

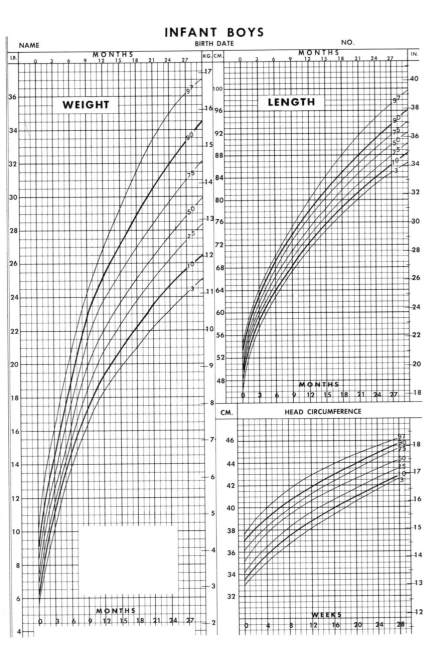

INFANT BOYS

NAME   BIRTH DATE   NO.

WEIGHT

LENGTH

HEAD CIRCUMFERENCE

MONTHS

WEEKS

221

GIRLS

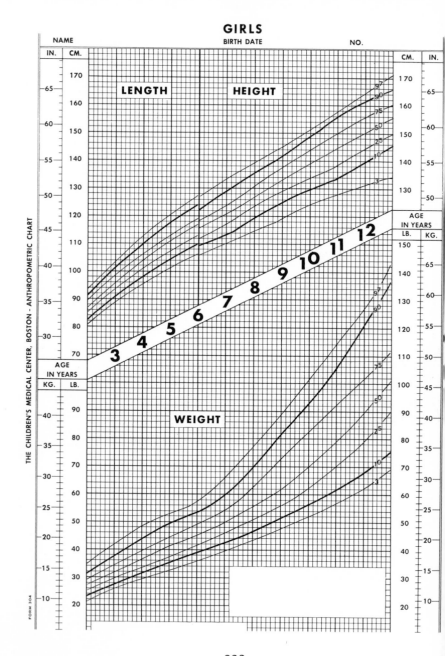

BOYS

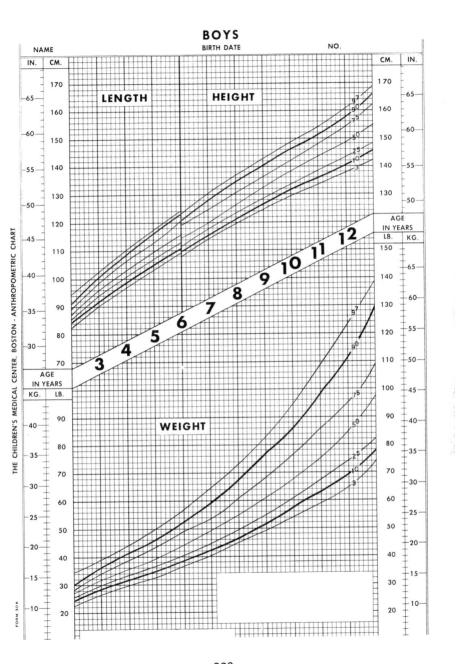

NAME   BIRTH DATE   NO.

LENGTH   HEIGHT

WEIGHT

AGE IN YEARS

THE CHILDREN'S MEDICAL CENTER, BOSTON - ANTHROPOMETRIC CHART

FORM 305

Index